APPROACHES TO DEATH AND DYING:

BIOETHICAL AND CULTURAL PERSPECTIVES

APPROACHES TO DEATH AND DYING:

BIOETHICAL AND CULTURAL PERSPECTIVES

Edited by
Marta Szabat
Jan Piasecki

Jagiellonian University Press

This publication is financed through the project No. N43/DBS/000187

Reviewer

dr hab. Agnieszka Kaczmarek, prof. UAM

Cover design: Paweł Sepielak

Cover photo: Tomasz Kowaluk, Pixabay

Cover text translated by Inter Lang & Text Translation Agency

ISBN 978-83-233-5055-2

ISBN 978-83-233-7282-0 (e-book)

JAGIELLONIAN
UNIVERSITY
PRESS

www.wuj.pl

Jagiellonian University Press
Editorial Offices: Michałowskiego 9/2, 31-126 Kraków, Poland
Phone: +48 12 663 23 80
Distribution: Phone: +48 12 631 01 97
Cell Phone: +48 506 006 674, e-mail: sprzedaz@wuj.pl
Bank: PEKAO SA, IBAN PL 80 1240 4722 1111 0000 4856 3325

Table of Contents

Cultural Studies on Death and Dying

Notes on Contributors

Barbara Bojdo, Jagiellonian University Medical College, Kraków, Poland.

Paulina Hornik, The Pontifical University of John Paul II in Kraków, Poland. ORCID: 0000-0002-6933-9075

Anna E. Kubiak, Institute of Philosophy and Sociology, Polish Academy of Science, Poland. ORCID: 0000-0002-9479-9700

Yael Lavi, School of Philosophy, Linguistics and Science Studies, Tel Aviv University, and Minerva Center for Interdisciplinary Studies of the End of Life, Tel Aviv University, Israel.

Łucja Lange, Sociology Institute, University of Lodz, and Literary Research Institute, Polish Academy of Sciences, Poland. ORCID: 0000-0002-2676-1022

Martyna Łaszewska-Hellriegel, Faculty of Law and Administration, University of Zielona Góra, Poland. ORCID: 0000-0002-2212-371X

Maria Onyszkiewicz, University of Warsaw, Department of Philosophy, Doctoral School of Humanities, Poland. ORCID: 0000-0002-7113-9064

Jan Piasecki, Department of Philosophy and Bioethics, Faculty of Health Sciences, Jagiellonian University Medical College, Kraków, Poland. ORCID: 0000-0003-1298-736X

Joanna Przybek-Mita, Institute of Health Sciences, College of Medical Sciences, University of Rzeszów, Poland. ORCID: 0000-0002-8403-5889

Zygmunt Pucko, Department of Philosophy and Bioethics, Faculty of Health Sciences, Jagiellonian University Medical College, Kraków, Poland. ORCID: 0000-0003-4859-4197

Valery Sokolchik, Belarusian Medical Academy of Postgraduate Education, Belarus. ORCID: 0000-0002-4975-4052

Marta Szabat, Department of Philosophy and Bioethics, Faculty of Health Sciences, Jagiellonian University Medical College, Kraków, Poland. ORCID: 0000-0001-5198-3842

Patrycja Zurzycka, Department of Clinical Nursing, Faculty of Health Sciences, Jagiellonian University Medical College, Kraków, Poland. ORCID: 0000-0002-2048-3711

Marta Szabat, Jan Piasecki

A Word from the Editors

The Encyclopedia Britannica defines death as "the total cessation of life processes that eventually occurs in all living organisms. The state of human death has always been obscured by mystery and superstition, and its precise definition remains controversial, differing according to culture and legal systems" (Encyclopedia Britannica 2021). Historically, the first definition of death in the field of medicine was proposed by the Ad Hoc Committee of Harvard Medical School to Examine the Definition of Brain Death (1968), which established four conditions necessary for declaring a person dead. These are as follows: (1) unreseptivity and unresponsivity; (2) no movements and breathing; (3) no reflexes—irreversible coma with the abolition of central nervous system activity; (4) flat electroencephalogram (Harvard. Definition 1968). Thirteen years later the President's Commission for the Study of Ethical Problems in Medicine and Biomedical and Behavioral Research in USA was set up to investigate similar issues. The commission published a report in which it proposed an alternative of two criteria for adjudicating death: "An individual who has sustained either (1) irreversible cessation of circulatory and respiratory functions, or (2) irreversible cessation of all functions of the entire brain, including the brain stem, is dead. The determination of death must be made in accordance with accepted medical standards" (Defining death 1981, p. 73). It is worth mentioning that the first country to incorporate a definition of brain death into its national law was Finland in 1971, doing so thus even before the "Defining death" report. Nowadays, in parallel with advances in mechanical ventilation, the development of transplantation procedures and life-support technology, countries all over the world have introduced their own definitions of brain death into their legislative or constitutional systems. In this context the most challenging distinction to be made is that between brain death and the other forms of brain damage that result in vegetative states. Another controversial issue is the criterion for determination of brain death in connection with the dead donor rule (Dalle Ave et al. 2020).

When it comes to individual and personal experiences of death and dying several highly sensitive ethical issues must be taken into account, such as decisions and choices in end-of-life (EOL) care, issues related to futile medical care, moral issues surrounding euthanasia and assisted dying. Additionally, the issue of communication between health care professionals (HCPs), patients and their families gives rise to several problems connected with the improper verbal and non-verbal language of HCPs, which can undermine the confidence of patients and their close relatives and friends in the accuracy of the patient's diagnosis, especially in highly vulnerable situations such as the decision to terminate causal treatment in order to begin palliative care (PC) or problems related to the issues of death and dying. In PC a pain treatment is provided at the holistic level and comprises various physical, psychological and spiritual aspects (Brown et al. 2016; Friedrichsdorf and Bruera 2018; Mok et al. 2010; Saunders et al. 1995; Saunders 2006). Hence, a personal approach to PC in each particular case is very demanding. Furthermore, when emphasizing the importance of PC, we should be aware that the purpose of such care is not actually to hasten death, which thus contrasts with euthanasia and medical assisted dying, which are more complex issues due to the greater autonomy of patients regarding the moment of their own death. However, in each country where euthanasia and assisted dying are legal PC continues to be provided until the moment of the patient's death. Accordingly, the patient's family also remains under PC both during the treatment of patient as well as in the bereavement period.

According to the medical anthropologist Byron Good, modern medicine construes the human body in an "illuminating and powerful" manner that allows us to control natural biological processes to a certain degree (1994). At the same time, medicine is not ideologically neutral and it imposes on us a scientific and reductionist understanding of a human being. This understanding leaves no place for individual, biographical experience and existential inquiries. However, as Good realizes, this does not mean that modern medicine neglects the spiritual or even soteriological dimensions of human life (Good 1994). While this may not be the case, however, it does colonize human experience and according to Good (1994, p. 86): "Sickness, death, and finitude are found in the corpse, in the human body. And salvation, or at least some partial representation of it, is present in the technical efficacy of medicine."

Medicine can "save" us, but the act of saving, in the case of a terminally ill patient, can only mean the prolongation of suffering. In such a situation death is perceived as liberation, and as Henk Ten Have and Jos Welie (2005) argue the euthanasia movement in the Netherlands was a protest directed against the authority of medicine and the prolongation of a barely biological existence. Euthanasia was conceived as a way out of the medicalization of death. Nonetheless Ten Have and Weile (2005) demonstrated that in actual fact decriminalization of this procedure transferred even more power into the hands of physicians. Once invited to a patient's death bed, a doctor not only helps to control the patient's pain and fear, but also decides when that patient has reached the moment of "unbearable suffering" and can be given a merciful death. As a consequence, in the Netherlands the *Uit Vrije Wil* (literally "out of free will") movement is now demanding the de-medicalization of euthanasia (Uit Vrije Will). Some might argue that this citizens' initiative is another symptom of a cultural shift in attitudes towards assisted dying (Lemmens 2018). Assisted dying is no longer seen as a last resort for a terminally ill patient experiencing unbearable physical pain and discomfort and seeking liberation from medicine. Nowadays, it is seen as a remedy for other kinds of suffering, as is epitomized by the Belgian case of Nathan Verhelst, who experienced mental suffering following unsuccessful gender reassignment surgery (Cook 2013). The medicalization of dying could have gone even further: a Belgian convicted murderer, Frank Van Den Bleeken requested euthanasia arguing that life imprisonment without adequate treatment put him in a position of "unbearable suffering." Although, his request for euthanasia was initially considered, it was eventually refused (Waterfield 2015). These cases seem to confirm Good's claim that medicine is colonizing human life, and since euthanasia or assisted suicide are considered to be medical procedures they are possible methods for dealing with human ailments that are deemed medical conditions.

However, assisted dying cannot exhaust all discussion surrounding EOL care (Saul 2012). In those countries where euthanasia or physician-assisted suicide is legal, only a small percentage of the dying request a doctor's assistance (Oregon Health Authority 2020). People do not want to die, but they do want to control the process of dying (Saul 2012). Moreover, it seems that not only physicians are equipped sufficiently to help humans with all matters concerning dying. Philosophy can bring some consolation, because philosophy is, according to the famous passage from Plato's Phaedo, the practice of dying. Moreover, Socrates contends that a philosopher who makes proper use of their reason can be persuaded by arguments that death is not dreadful, because there is an afterworld. Nowadays, we are rather inclined to say that death limits reason. But it does mean that our reason, wit and creativity cannot help us deal with the ultimate issues of life, as is also demonstrated in this volume.

This monograph broadens and deepens our understand of several aspects of death and dying. The authors discuss such issues as euthanasia and assisted dying in both Europe and in USA, an advance care planning, the importance of family support in the case of oncological or long-term diseases, as well as patient and parental autonomy in EOL care. Additionally, EOL issues are examined in the context of biopolitics, the bioeconomy, and the problem of posthumous harm. Furthermore, from a cultural perspective, the concept of "the cancertainment" adds new meaning to the cultural perception of cancer as a way of disseminating knowledge and reducing tension between those who suffer due to cancer and those who have only an exaggerated idea of the disease. Our understanding of death is also expanded through reflections on various artistic visions of death and dying, such as Frida Kahlo's canvases which reveal her own internal and external landscapes of life in "living death" as well as the iconography of death in European art from Antiquity up to modern times.

References

Brown E.M., Thorn C., Cowell D. 2016. Compassionate extubation in the home: It takes a team. *Journal of Pain and Symptom Management* 51(2): 337–338.

Cook M. 2013. Belgian euthanased after botched sex-change operation. *BioEdge. Bioethics news from around the world.* Available at: https://www.bioedge.org/bioethics/bioethics_article/10707. Accessed: 22.08.2021.

Dalle Ave A.L., Sulmasy D.P., Bernat J.L. 2020. The ethical obligation of the dead donor rule. *Medicine, Health Care and Philosophy* 23: 43–50.

Defining death. 1981. Defining death, a report on the medical, legal, and ethical issues in the determination of Heath. President's Commission for the Study of Ethical Problems in Medicine and Biomedical and Behavioral Research. Available at: https://repository.library.georgetown.edu/bitstream/handle/10822/559345/defining_death.pdf?sequence=1&isAllowed=y. Accessed: 27.03.2021.

Encyclopedia Britannica. 2021. *Death.* Available at: https://www.britannica.com/science/death. Accessed: 27.03.2021.

Friedrichsdorf S.J., Bruera E. 2018. Delivering pediatric palliative care: From denial, palliphobia, pallilalia to palliactive. *Children. Special Issue of Pediatric Palliative Care* 5(9): 120.

Good B.J. 1994. *Medicine, Rationality, and Experience. An Anthropological Perspective.* Cambridge: Cambridge University Press.

Harvard. Definition. 1968. A Definition of irreversible coma report of the ad hoc Committee of Harvard Medical School to examine the definition of brain death. *JAMA* 205(6): 337–340. Available at: https://jamanetwork.com/journals/jama/article-abstract/340177. Accessed: 27.03.2021.

Lemmens T. 2018. Charter scrutiny of Canada's medical assistance in dying law and the shifting landscape of Belgian and Dutch euthanasia practice. *Supreme Court Law Review (2nd Series)* 85: 459–544.

Mok E., Lau K., Lam W., Chan L., Ng J., Chan K. 2010. Health-care professionals' perspective on hope in the palliative care setting. *Journal of Palliative Medicine* 13(7): 877–883.

Oregon Health Authority. 2020. *Oregon Death with Dignity Act. Data Summary 2019.* Available at: https://www.oregon.gov/oha/PH/PROVIDERPARTNERRESOURCES/EVALUATIONRESEARCH/DEATHWITHDIGNITYACT/Documents/year22.pdf. Accessed: 21.04.2021.

Saul P. 2012. Let's talk about dying. *TedTalk*. Available at: https://www.ted.com/talks/peter_saul_let_s_talk_about_dying?language=en. Accessed: 23.04.2021.

Saunders C. 2006. *Selected Writings*. Oxford, New York: Oxford University Press.

Saunders C., Baines M., Dunlop R. 1995. *Living with Dying. A Guide to Palliative Care*. Oxford: Oxford University Press.

Ten Have H., Welie J. 2005. Death and Medical Power: An Ethical Analysis of Dutch Euthanasia Practice: An Ethical Analysis of Dutch Euthanasia Practice. New York: McGraw-Hill Education.

Uit Vrije Wil. Available at: http://uitvrijewil.nu/. Accessed: 23.04.2021.

Waterfield B. 2015. Belgian serial rapist will not be euthanised. *Telegraph*, 6 January. Available at: https://www.telegraph.co.uk/news/worldnews/europe/belgium/11327541/Belgian-serial-rapist-will-not-be-euthanised-as-planned.html. Accessed: 23.04.2021.

Legal and Ethical Aspects of Patient Autonomy

Martyna Łaszewska-Hellriegel

Deciding Life and Death: Euthanasia in Europe. Ethical and Regulatory Implications

Abstract

The aim of this chapter is to present and categorize the ethical aspects of euthanasia and assisted suicide. For this purpose, the authors applied the four main moral principles of bioethics, namely: patient autonomy, beneficence, utility, and justice. These are suitable principles because they enable reflection on the practice of euthanasia not only within the scope of individual rights and needs, but also in the context of social implications. In fact, many bioethical issues arise from conflicts inherent within these basic principles. This approach will be supplemented with an analysis of a recent significant court decision on euthanasia and assisted suicide in Europe.

Keywords: euthanasia, assisted suicide, autonomy, beneficence, utility, justice

Introduction

In his book *The World Until Yesterday* the American geographer, historian, anthropologist and ornithologist Jared Diamond envisions societies in which children should, and in certain circumstances do, neglect, abandon or kill their parents (Diamond 2012, p. 214). In his opinion, this happens in two kinds of society: among nomadic hunter gatherers who must move camp from time to time in order to maintain their supply of food, and in arctic and desert regions where severe food shortages occur periodically. In both situations, we see scarce resources and the perceived burden of elderly parents to society as the motivating factors. Furthermore, Diamond identifies five different ways of killing, arranging them in a sequence of increasingly direct action starting from the most passive method to the most active (Diamond 2012, pp. 215–217). The most passive approach is neglect (giving little food, ignoring needs, etc.), which is something akin to passive euthanasia (not necessarily voluntary). The second approach is to intentionally abandon an old or sick person or to bring an old person to the forest and leave them to walk off and never be seen again—this could be qualified as active euthanasia (either voluntary or not). The third method involves an old person choosing or being encouraged to commit suicide, for example by "jumping off a cliff, going out to sea, or seeking death in battle," which can be qualified as assisted suicide. The fourth method can be described either as assisted suicide or as killing the victim with the latter's cooperation, by strangling, stabbing or burying them. The final method is to kill the victim violently without the victim's cooperation or consent (Diamond 2012, pp. 215–217). In modern societies, where the same scarcity of resources cannot be said to exist, we can still observe different forms of legal voluntary euthanasia or assisted suicide performed out of mercy as well as cases of active euthanasia, both of which are a cause of controversy. The main problem with these "methods of dying" is the question of whether we have the "right to die" and, if so, how to make sure that the decision to die is taken autonomously. Different countries try to put forward their own rules regulating those situations in which euthanasia would be possible so as to ensure that it does not morph into killing. However these rules do not always work in certain complicated scenarios written by life itself. The aim of this chapter is to present and categorize the ethical aspects of euthanasia and assisted suicide. The four main moral principles of bioethics will be used for this purpose: patient autonomy, beneficence, utility, and justice. They are suitable for this task as they enable reflection on the practice of euthanasia not only within the scope of individual rights and needs, but also with regard to social implications (Beauchamp and Childress 1994, p. 7). In fact, many bioethical issues arise from conflicts inherent within these basic principles. This approach will be supplemented with an analysis of a recent significant court decision on euthanasia and assisted suicide in Europe.

Active euthanasia *versus* passive euthanasia and assisted suicide

For the purposes of clarity, euthanasia can be characterized as directly or indirectly bringing about the death of another person for the latter person's sake (Foot 1977, p. 85). The term derives from the Greek word meaning *good death* and evokes the idea that causing or contributing to somebody's end may be good for that person. Many philosophers uphold the view that there are two forms of euthanasia (Vaughn 2010, p. 528). Active euthanasia is said to involve performing an action that directly causes someone to die as a result of what most people think of as a mercy killing. Passive euthanasia is enabling someone to die by refraining from doing something that would prolong their life. This conceptual boundary between active and passive euthanasia is crucial for assessing the morality of euthanasia. Letting a patient die is sometimes morally acceptable while being directly involved in killing them is always wrong. The former practice is legal in some countries provided certain conditions are met; the latter is mostly illegal, with the exception of a few countries (e.g., Belgium and Holland). Euthanasia can be considered morally wrong or right and this does not depend solely on the active versus passive divide. If euthanasia in some form is morally permissible, its permissibility must be linked to the patient's consent. Euthanasia can be voluntary, non-voluntary, or involuntary.

Voluntary euthanasia refers to situations in which a competent patient voluntarily requests or agrees to euthanasia, communicating their wishes either while in full possession of their faculties or through instructions to be followed if they become incapacitated (if they fall into a persistent vegetative state). Patients specify what is to be done in cases of incapacity by expressing an advance directive (commonly a living will or a document designating a surrogate, or proxy, to act on their behalf).

Non-voluntary euthanasia is performed when patients are unable to choose death for themselves and have not previously disclosed their preferences (incompetent adults, infants and children). In these situations, the patient's family physicians, or other legally designated persons decide for the patient.

Involuntary euthanasia involves situations where a person's death is brought about against his or her will or without asking their consent while they are still competent to decide. It is illegal and considered morally wrong. It is therefore left out of the moral debate, except perhaps in the case of slippery-slope arguments to the effect that voluntary or non-voluntary euthanasia will inevitably become involuntary (Vaughn 2010, p. 528).

In a physician-assisted suicide, a patient takes his or her own life with the aid of a physician. In a typical scenario, the patient asks the physician for help in their efforts to commit suicide, and the physician assists the patient by prescribing a lethal dose of drugs or by explaining to them particular methods of suicide; it is the patient—not the physician—who performs the final act that results in death. By way of contrast, in cases involving active euthanasia the physician performs the final act. Many argue that this difference in the ultimate cause of death implies a difference in terms of moral responsibility (Nesbitt 1995, pp.101–105).

Ethical questions. Autonomy

Autonomy refers to a person's rational capacity for self-governance or self-determination—the ability to control one's own life and make choices for oneself. The principle of autonomy rests on the individual's autonomy being fully respected (Vaughn 2010, p. 9). In medical ethics, respecting a patient's autonomy includes respecting individual decisions when it comes to requesting or refusing medical treatment. Formally, this principle has been applied in relation the notion of informed consent. Without such consent from the patient, no medical intervention can be performed. Respect for the patient's autonomy is not only ensured by accepting their decisions regarding the acceptance or refusal of a medical treatment. Informed consent should also be accompanied by detailed advice and a well-considered assessment process, which in its ideal form comprises shared decision-making, including open conversations between the patient and the doctor. In this model, the patient is not only given time to learn all the relevant information from the doctor, but the patient's needs and preferences should also be carefully and adequately considered. The professional co-responsibility of the doctor for the final decision is also important (Krones and Richter 2008, p. 818). Conflicts between respecting a patient's autonomy and a physician's duty of beneficence usually give rise to the issue of paternalism, which can be defined as the act of overriding a person's actions or making decisions on their behalf and for their own good. Major ethical theories take diverging stands on paternalism. In the case of act-utilitarianism, the rightness of an act depends on the good maximized, according to the rules governing different categories of actions. On the grounds of act utilitarianism, a physician may judge that it is morally permissible to lie to a patient about certain beneficial treatment in order to overcome a patient's refusal to be treated. Philosophers who follow John Stuart Mill's lead, however, would reject such paternalism. Mill believed that the principle of utility indicates profound respect for a person's self-determination and declares that no one can impede an individual's liberty except in order to prevent harm to others. As Mill said, "a person cannot rightfully be compelled to do or forbear because it will be better for him to do so, because it will make him happier, because, in the opinion of others, to do so would be wise, or even right" (Mill 1859, p. 18). In this understanding, people should be allowed to choose what can be done to their own bodies. This implies the right to reject treatment, and on the other hand to the right to informed consent. Kantian ethics also dismisses paternalism. The means-end of the categorical imperative calls for respect for the rights and autonomy of individuals. This principle requires physicians to accept a patient's decision to refuse treatment, even if they believe such treatment is life-saving (Vaughn 2010, p. 9).

How much self-determination is there? A case study in Holland

The right to self-determination is our primal right derived from natural rights and inscribed into all major constitutions and human rights conventions around the world. The right to die is based on this principle. The problem is that it is not always easy to decide if consent given to end a life was autonomous, thereby making euthanasia or assisted suicide ethically justified. Where should we draw the line between euthanasia and homicide? What can we do to protect patients from the will of others? How can we ensure that the will of people with dementia is respected? To answer these questions let us look at a recent decision of a criminal court in The Hague dating from September 11, 2019.

The criminal court found a doctor not guilty of killing a woman with late-stage Alzheimer's (in this chapter the woman is referred to as Ms. A). In the early stages of her illness, Ms. A had repeatedly stated that if her illness progressed under no circumstances would she allow herself to be placed in a nursing home and instead would wish her life to end (De Rechtspraak Den Haag, 11.9.2019). On April 21, 2020, the Supreme Court (de Hoge Raad 21.4.2020) upheld the lower court's verdict of not guilty and overturned disciplinary proceedings against doctor. The court also issued an opinion on the fundamental issues regarding the euthanasia of patients with severe dementia (Hoge Raad, 21.4.2020, 19/04910).

On October 2, 2012, and after conducting a specialist examination Ms. A, who was 70 or 71 at the time, was diagnosed with early-stage Alzheimer's disease. Her mother had also suffered from Alzheimer's disease and had spent many years in a nursing home. Ms. A described being "seriously traumatized" by witnessing her mother's suffering and did not want to follow the same path under any circumstances. On October 20, 2012, she signed several documents including a refusal to consent to certain treatment and a request for her life to be terminated should she reach a state of intolerable suffering with no prospect of recovery. She also signed a statement explicitly declaring that that her wishes should be respected in the more distant future. Under no circumstances did she want to be placed in a nursing home for dementia patients. Euthanasia would take place the moment she was no longer able to live at home with her husband. According to her family physician Ms. A provided a clear and coherent justification for her statement. In January 2013, in a letter to the same doctor, a specialist confirmed that the patient had made her decisions in a *compos mentis* state. In 2015, Ms. A repeated her will in writing as well as her categorical refusal to be admitted to a nursing home. She supplemented her statement with the following sentence "euthanasia may be performed at my request." From July 2015, her condition deteriorated significantly. Eventually, she had to be admitted to a nursing home, where the defendant worked as a doctor specializing in geriatric diseases. In a conversation in January 2016, the family doctor stated that she was no longer capable of independent judgment and also did not know what termination of life meant. However, when asked, she said that she did not want to die at that moment. On March 8 and March 10, when asked directly and repeatedly whether she wanted to die, Ms. A gave negative answers ("not now"). In these conversations, however, Ms. A was very confused. In the nursing home, it was noted that Ms. A was almost constantly in a state of agitation, restlessness, stress, anxiety, sadness, anger and panic. The accused physician consulted with the family doctor, the husband and the daughter of Ms. A, as well as with a psychologist and an end-of-life counselor. Two other physicians independently concluded that the patient's compliance with the instructions to end her life was in accordance with the legal rules of care. On April 22, 2016, the defendant first placed a sedative in Ms. A's coffee after which he administered a lethal injection. Ms. A had to be held down during the lethal injection because she tried to unrestrain herself.

The Dutch legal context

Section 293(1) of the Dutch Criminal Code (NL-CC) prohibits killing on demand. However, the punishment for intentional homicide is much less severe if it is committed at the express and serious request of the person killed. The provision contains an exception clause that excludes punishment (sec. 293(2) NL-CC) if a physician acts in compliance with a certain duty of care. The duties of care are laid down in sec. 2(1) of the Termination of Life on Request and Assisted Suicide Act (ToLaAS). In accordance with this statute a physician must:

(a) have come to the conclusion that the patient's request is voluntary and been properly considered;
(b) be convinced that the patient's condition is hopeless and his/her suffering is unbearable;
(c) have informed the patient of his or her medical condition and life prospects (prognosis);
(d) have come to the conclusion, together with the patient, that there is no other acceptable solution given the patient's situation;
(e) have consulted at least one other independent physician who has examined the patient and provided a written opinion on the criteria of care stated in subparagraphs (a) to (d);
(f) terminated the life of the patient or assisted in his/her suicide while maintaining due medical care.

Section 2(2) of the ToLaAS refers to the fact that a request for termination of life may be granted if the patient who has reached the age of sixteen is unable to express his or her will, but who, prior to the occurrence of this condition, could have been considered capable of acting in his or her interests and has made a written declaration expressing their desire for treatment to terminate their life.

The first part of the opinion contained in the verdict of acquittal addresses the question of whether the act should be classified as homicide or homicide on demand (sec. 293(1) NL-CC). The public prosecutor's office had expressed the view that it was imperative that Ms. A had articulated her wish to die to the defendant close to the time of the fatal act. Since this had not happened, and Ms. A even tried to unrestrain herself, it was a case of homicide. The court did not agree. It was sufficient that the previous statements of the patient's will were clear, consistent and formulated while Ms. A still had the capacity for independent judgment regarding the termination of her life. From sec. 2(2) of the ToLaAS, it follows that termination of life is possible on the basis of a written statement, if the patient is no longer able to verbally express his or her will. The court pointed out that legislative interpretations cite as examples not only coma states, but also severe dementia. The court checked if the defendant (the physician) had not been obliged under sec. 293(2) NL-CC to question Ms. A again and obtain an oral confirmation that the wish set out in writing still existed on April 22, 2016. The court rejected the existence of such a duty to ask such a question in those circumstances, in line with sec. 2(2) of the ToLaAS. The case only required application of the rules set out in sec. 2(1) of the ToLaAS. The normally existing requirement of informed consent and counseling is no longer necessary if patients are not able to express their coherent will. The ruling emphasizes that physicians, in addition to a patient's declaration of intent made in a state of sound mind, must also determine whether the patient's condition is hopeless and the suffering unbearable. It is important to point out that a diagnosis of severe dementia is not sufficient in itself. In the case under discussion, the assumption that Ms. A was experiencing severe mental suffering was based on the behavior and he recognizably desperate emotional state. The Hoge Raad upheld the acquittal and issued some general guidelines on euthanasia in cases of dementia. Euthanasia on request may be performed providing that the patient's written request explicitly refers to situations in which advanced dementia makes it impossible for the patient to express their own will. Beyond this specific case, it is important to note that there may be circumstances in which a patient's current behavior indicates that their condition does not correspond to their state at the time they gave their previous instructions. The Hoge Raad also stressed the fact that extreme suffering must be carefully determined. Even though in legislative history this requirement has primarily referred to physical suffering, it is possible that severe dementia may lead to unbearable suffering. The procedural requirements for such an assessment were also tightened: in the case of patients with dementia, two independent physicians are needed to confirm that the legal requirements for euthanasia have been met. With regard to the implementation of these rules, the court judged that it is permissible to sedate patients if irrational and unpredictable behavior is to be expected.

Self-determination in the context of dementia

Two questions remain to be considered in light of the opinion presented by the Dutch courts: the first relates to whether an earlier, self-determined desire becomes irrelevant if the person in the state of severe dementia subsequently behaves in a manner that could be interpreted as a change in the way he or she evaluates the situation. Why was Ms. A's expressed verbal wish "not now" ignored and not interpreted as binding?

The Dutch ruling states that there may be circumstances in which an express and explicit desire to commit assisted suicide or euthanasia may conflict with later verbal or behavioral expressions, allowing for the conclusion that a person's current circumstances do not correspond to the circumstances in which they originally made the request. With regard to the specific case in question, this did not matter because there were no indications that Ms. A felt her actual living conditions in the nursing home to be different to those she had anticipated. Nevertheless, the short legal note is interesting, because such cases can occur. Of practical importance is the question of whether the medical treatment specified in a patient's statement may be discontinued if the patient, who in the meantime develops dementia, shows signs of sustained zest for life and well-being. This leads to the fundamental question of whether it depends solely on the patient's reflected will, which presupposes an ability to make judgments, or also on the expression of the patient's current state of mind—often called "natural will," or, more appropriately, signs of current desires (Jox 2006, pp. 69, 81). In the case of medical and nursing ethics, when it comes to the question of appropriate treatment for dementia patients, it is easy to justify that care and respect should be linked to bodily signs (Fuchs 2018, pp. 48–49). It is more difficult to evaluate the fundamental decisions that go beyond everyday needs. Philosophical and medical ethics offer contradictory positions. Some authors give priority to self-determined expressions of will over past anticipations (Dworkin 1993, p. 226). According to another view, in the event of an obvious conflict with the current state or situation, an earlier decision should not be implemented, even if this earlier decision met the cognitive-mental requirements for self-determination (Cohen-Almagor 2016, p. 74). Anyone who assumes that an earlier self-determined disposition for euthanasia or termination of treatment is overridden by the current state of a person with dementia must address the issue of what constitutes conclusive evidence of changed wishes. Misinterpretations are to be expected: observers tend to transfer meanings onto the behavior of people with dementia even if there are other physiological and psychological explanations (Jox 2006, p. 78). Critical reports on the Dutch case highlighted the fact that in 2016, Ms. A. addressed such phrases as "not now" to her family doctor and nursing home doctor when they tried to explain to her what euthanasia was (which she no longer knew). Did these verbalizations have no significance because of her lost ability to communicate? Is it reasonable to assume that Ms. A felt that the questioning and insistence of the physicians was a stressful and unpleasant experience, and, as a consequence, responded with evasive words? Or was it her intention to say "not now" to euthanasia? This is a mystery we will never know. The only indication of a change in the wishes of a person with dementia would be a change in their overall behavior indicating in a reasonably consistent manner that their earlier self-determined disposition was based on a misjudgment. Ms. A was not happy in the nursing home, but at the same time she also did not appear to want to be administered a lethal injection. Perhaps the wishes of her family and doctors were being honored instead of her own?

Ethical questions. Beneficence

The principle of beneficence constitutes the very essence of morality—or is very close to it. In its broadest meaning, it states that we should do good to others and avoid doing them harm. These two injunctions—to both do good and avoid harm—are distinct. The former—active beneficence—enjoins us to advance the welfare of others and prevent harm being done to them; the latter—nonmaleficence—asks us not to, intentionally or unintentionally, inflict harm on others (Vaughn 2010, p. 10).

The principle of beneficence lies at the heart of many disputes because the obligation to help or not to harm subjects often appears to be in conflict with the aim of euthanasia (Breen 2003, p. 186). One of the central tasks of a doctor when treating a patient is to achieve a balance between harming and benefiting the patient. Both principles are therefore essential components of the medical duty of care and consequently will be discussed together. The decision as to whether euthanasia may be considered ethically justifiable is discussed in the literature mainly from the perspective of two principles: the principle of autonomy (already discussed above) and the principle of beneficence or mercy. If we are in a position to relieve the extreme suffering of another without any excessive cost to ourselves, we have a duty to do so. To refuse would be cruel, inhumane and wrong. The argument would run like this: If a competent, hopelessly ill patient in unrelieved pain requests assistance so that they can be put out of their misery, we may have the duty to bring about his death. Brock says that for patients not receiving life-sustaining treatment (where passive euthanasia applies) active euthanasia or assisted suicide may be the only release from their "otherwise prolonged suffering and agony" (Brock 1992, pp. 19–21). In such circumstances, active euthanasia or assisted suicide is sometimes better than passive alternatives, for withholding or withdrawing treatment from a dying patient in unspeakable pain may only prolong their agony. Death may not cause harm, but allowing active euthanasia or assisted suicide will inevitably lead to heinous extensions or perversions of original practices. Among the typical concerns is the fear that legalization will quickly lead from active voluntary euthanasia to active non-voluntary euthanasia and even to outright involuntary forms of killing. There is also the danger that physicians or families will start pushing unwilling or unsure patients towards assisted suicide or voluntary euthanasia, or that physicians and nurses will become increasingly willing to administer lethal injections to people who are elderly, mentally ill, uninsured, or disabled. Policy in this area definitely lies on a "slippery slope" (Gay-Williams 2004, p. 710).

The German Constitutional Court on assisted suicide services

A recent judgement of the German Federal Constitutional Court—*Bundes Verfassungsgericht* (BVerfG) from 26.2.2020 (BVerfG, 26.2.20, phr. 1–343) declared that criminalisation of assisted suicide services was unconstitutional. The court acknowledged that the general right of personality (Art. 2(1) in conjunction with Art. 1(1) of the Basic Law, *Grundgesetz*—GG) includes the right to self-determined death. This right covers the freedom to take one's own life and, if this is the case, allows for assistance from third persons. In cases where, in the exercise of this right, an individual decides to end their own life, having reached this decision based on how they personally define quality of life and meaningful existence, their decision must, in principle, be respected by the state and society as an act of autonomous self-determination (BVerfG, 26.2.20, phr. 1–343). For these reasons, the Second Senate of the Federal Constitutional Court held s that the prohibition of assisted suicide services set out in §217 of the German Criminal Code (*Strafgesetzbuch*—StGB) violates Basic Law and is void. The Court found that, in practice, this prohibition effectively vitiates any possibility that the individual concerned can chose assisted suicide and die in dignity if they wish to do so. It does not follow from this judgment that the legislator is barred under constitutional law from imposing any rules on suicide assistance. However, when enacting legislative provisions, it has to ensure that sufficient space remains for the individual to exercise their right to a self-determined death and to pursue and carry out their decision to end their life on their own terms.

This court's decision triggered a debate on how to protect people from non-autonomous decisions. Sick and old people in particular can feel under pressure. The feeling of being a burden on others is a major factor in the decision-making process (Grunert 2020, p. 2). Furthermore, the legislator anticipates the possibility that professional assisted suicide services could lead to "societal normalisation" of assisted suicide and euthanasia. As a result, assisted suicide could become recognised as a normal way of ending life, especially for elderly and ill persons. Countries with liberal laws on assisted suicide and euthanasia have experienced a steady increase in assisted suicide and voluntary euthanasia (Grunert 2020, p. 2). In Switzerland, the number of assisted suicides doubled between 2009 and 2014 following liberalisation of the laws in that country (Pereira 2011, p. 38). Assisted suicide is so often offered as an option in Dutch nursing homes that older people from border regions try to secure places in German nursing homes to escape constant nagging (Grunert 2020, p. 2). In addition, deaths from assisted suicide in the American state of Oregon are economically justified. In the case of some incurable illnesses, treatment costs are not covered by the patient's insurance, while the costs of lethal injection are included (Grunert 2020, p. 2). The increase in cases of assisted suicides and euthanasia is not necessarily proof of "societal normalisation" or the existence of social pressure endangering autonomy. It can also be explained by greater acceptance in society of assisted suicide and therefore a "strengthening of the right to self-determination, or growing awareness that the terms of one's own death need not invariably be accepted as fate beyond one's control" (BVerfG, 26.2.2020, no. 3(2)). Even so, the legislator faces considerable pressure to draft provisions stipulating that professional assisted suicide services should not place the principle of self-determination at risk. Bearing in mind the growing financial strain on long-term care and healthcare systems, this fact is especially true where healthcare and long-term care services struggle to meet demands. These developments may instil in some individuals a fear of loss of self-determination and could thus encourage decisions to commit suicide. As was mentioned above and confirmed by various studies, a common motive for seeking suicide assistance is the desire not to burden relatives or third parties (McPherson et al. 2007, p. 9).

Ethical questions. Utility

According to the principle of utility, we must ensure the most favorable balance of good over bad (or benefit over harm) for all parties concerned (Vaughn 2010, p. 11). This principle acknowledges that in the real world we cannot always act simply to benefit others or avoid doing them harm. Often, we cannot do good to people without at the same time acting to their detriment in some way, or we cannot help everyone who needs to be helped, or we cannot help some people without also hurting or neglecting others. In such situations, the principle of utility states that we should do what yields the best overall outcome—maximum good and minimum evil for everyone concerned. The utility principle is thus a supplement to, and not a substitute for, the principles of autonomy, beneficence and justice.

A physician must decide whether euthanasia or assisted suicide is right for the patient. This kind of decision is one of the hardest to take, since once the decision is made in favor of euthanasia, the outcome cannot be changed. The primary goal then is to design a policy that would ensure that such decisions are autonomous.

How do we make sure that a decision is autonomous—is this an illusion?

Appropriate policy planning in this area is a question that occupies many lawyers and doctors seeking an ethically justified solution. Eight researchers from the Universities of Halle, Augsburg and Munich recently drew up their own proposal (Dorneck et al. 2021, pp. 1–87). These legal scholars and medical ethicists, including Henning Rosenau and Jens Kersten, not only want to fill the gaps left by the aforementioned ruling of the German Federal Constitutional Court (BVerfG, 26.2.2020), but also reorganize the system of euthanasia as a whole. The draft proposal also contains suggested provisions regulating the termination of treatment and living wills, for example, as well as guidelines for suicide prevention programs. Following the Constitutional Court's decision, the proposal clarifies the fact that every person has the right to end his or her own life, provided that he or she acts in a freely responsible manner. The prevention of such suicides should be forbidden, while participation should be permissible. This reflects the current state of the law in Germany, because since suicide is not an illegal act, assisting it cannot be punishable either. For physicians, however, the situation is more difficult, as assisted suicide is prohibited in ten of the seventeen professional codes of medical practice in force in the country. Academics argue that doctors should be allowed to freely participate in assisted suicide, i.e. by prescribing a lethal dose of certain anesthetics under certain conditions. The person wishing to die must first be given detailed advice and be informed of palliative medical options. In addition, an independent commission must issue an expert's opinion on the voluntary nature of the person's will to die. Comprehensive documentation is also required (Grunert and Bubrowski 2021, p. 3).

Ethical questions. Justice

In the broadest sense of the term, justice dictates that people should receive what is fair or what is their due. Most of us seem to develop an idea of what justice entails in various life circumstances, even if we are not able to express what precisely it is. In philosophy, there are different understandings of justice rooted in different philosophical ideas. In the context of euthanasia and assisted suicide, philosophers coincidentally adopt different views on active euthanasia and assisted suicide depending on how they define the good to be maximized, whether the focus of their ethics is acts or rules, and how much importance they assign to self-determination (Vallentyne 2012, p. 152). *Classic utilitarianism* defines good as happiness and as a consequence evaluates questions in terms of how much happiness different activities might yield for the persons involved. From this viewpoint, euthanasia or assisted suicide might be justified in the case of someone suffering terrible and unavoidable pain. Bringing life and suffering to an end would produce the greatest net happiness. A different approach is proposed by another school of utilitarian thinking called *preference utilitarianism*. which accepts the view that the correct actions are those that please more people generally. According to preference utilitarianism, killing is immoral when it stops someone from fulfilling their own preferences, but killing can be deemed a good deed (as in the case of euthanasia) (Singer 2003, pp. 526–41). There are also some critics who claim that a general policy of authorized killing will gradually take society down a more catastrophic path. The outcomes to be avoided are a substantial increase in non-voluntary or involuntary euthanasia, an erosion of respect for the medical profession, and a weakening of society's abhorrence of homicide (Blackorby et al. 1999, p. 544).

The natural law view in Roman Catholicism condemns both active and passive euthanasia, although this condemnation comes with qualifications. Directly intending to bring about a person's death in order to put an end to their misery is forbidden, but the doctrine of double effect permits actions that have unintended but fatal results. Catholic teaching does not specify any obligation to use every means possible to prolong a person's life in every case.

What is clear in Kantian theory is that suicide is forbidden because it treats people as mere things and destroys personhood. In Kant's view competent individuals may not be killed or allowed to die. However, it is not clear what Kant's position would be if people were no longer viewed as people because they have fallen into a permanent vegetative state. Should we respect a person's request that they be kept alive no matter what the price—or should we refrain from voluntary euthanasia so as to allow them to die with dignity?

Conclusions

Euthanasia and assisted suicide will continue to raise many ethical issues. Accordingly, the ethical questions and problems that arise from a decision to terminate life are complex and wide-ranging. The suffering caused by pain and our free will to decide whether and when to end our lives legitimizes voluntary euthanasia and assisted suicide. Considering the many serious ethical problems that arise when assessing whether self-determination is maintained, especially in the case of patients with dementia and patients who cannot express their will, we should establish procedural rules for verifying self-determination. These are of key importance because severe and unavoidable suffering is not a sufficient condition on its own distinguishing self-determined decisions from those made by others. An effective system of review should include an individual primary review comprising examinations and interviews with the person wishing to die, with an ex-post assurance to check whether there are any deficiencies in the primary review system. Such procedural safeguards are provided for under Dutch law (Berghmans and Widdershoven 2012, p. 39). We could think of a number of conceivable improvements, for example in the form of psychological or psychiatric expertise provided when drafting a patient decree in the event of dementia, and giving a second opinion as early as when the written request to die is first made (and not only when the request is implemented) (Miller et al. 2019, pp. 84, 87). The law should permit euthanasia on the one hand, so as to do justice to a person's right to self-determined dying. On the other hand, however, it should counteract external influences so as to provide protection for patients.

References

Beauchamp T.L., Childress J.F. 1994. *Principles of Biomedical Ethics*. New York: Oxford University Press.

Berghmans R., Widdershoven G. 2012. Euthanasia in the Netherlands: Consultation and review. *King's Law Journal* 23: 109–118.

Brock D. 1992. Voluntary active euthanasia. *Hastin Center Reports* 22(2), March/April: 19–21.

Breen K.J. 2003. Misconduct in medical research: Whose responsibility? *International Medicine Journal* 33: 186–191.

Blackorby Ch., Bossert W., Donaldson D. 1999. Utilitarianism and the theory of justice. In *Handbook of Social Choice and Welfare*, ed. K. Arrow, K. Amartya Sen, K. Suzumura, 543–596. Amsterdam: Elsevier.

Cohen-Almagor R. 2016. First do no harm: Euthanasia of patients with dementia in Belgium. *The Journal of Medicine and Philosophy* 41(1): 74–89.

Diamond J. 2012. *The World until Yesterday. What Can we Learn from Traditional Societies?* New York: Viking.

Dworkin R. 1994. *Life's Dominion: An Argument about Abortion, Euthanasia, and Individual Freedom*. New York: Vintage Books.

Dorneck C., Gassner U.M., Kersten J., Lindner F.J., Linoh K.Ph., Lorenz H., Henning Rosenau H., Schmidt B. 2021. *Gesetz zur Gewährleistung selbstbestimmten Sterbens und zur Suizidprävention, Augsburg-Münchner-Hallescher-Entwurf (AMHE-SterbehilfeG)*. Tübingen: Mohr Siebeck.

Foot F. 1977. Euthanasia. *Philosophy and Public Affairs* 6(2): 85–112.

Fuchs T. 2018. Leiblichkeit und personale Identität in der Demen. *DZPhil* 66(1): 48–61.

Gay-Williams J. 2004. The wrongfulness of euthanasia in intervention and reflection. In *Basics Isuess in Medical Ethics*, ed. R. Mundson. California: Belemont.

Grunert M. 2020. So emotional wie selten. *Frankfurter Allgemeine Zeitung*, 17.02.2020.

Grunert M., Bubrowski H. 2021. Rechtsunsicherheit auf dem letzten weg. *Frankfurter Allgemeine Zeitung*, 05.02.2021. Available at: https://www.faz.net/aktuell/politik/inland/bundesverfassungsgericht-entscheidet-ueber-sterbehilfe-17183462-p2.html. Accessed: 11.02.2021.

Jox R.J. 2006. Der „natürliche Wille" als Entscheidungskriterium: rechtliche, handlungstheoretische und ethische Aspekte. In *Entscheidungen am Lebensende in der modernen Medizin: Ethik, Recht, Ökonomie und Klinik*, eds. J. Schildmann, U. Fahr, J. Vollmann, 73–89. Münster: LIT-Verlag.

Krones T., Richter G. 2008. Ärztliche Verantwortung. Das Arzt-Patient-Verhältnis. *Bundesgesundheitsblatt Gesundheitsforschung Gesundheitsschutz* 51: 818–826.

McPherson Ch., Keith J., Wilson G., Murray M.A. 2007. Feeling like a burden to others: A systematic review focusing on the end of life. *Paliative medicine* 21(7).

Miller D.G., Dresser R., Kim S. 2019. Advance euthanasia directives: A controversial case and its ethical implications. *Journal of Medical Ethics* 45(2): 84–89.

Mill J.S. 1859. *On Liberty*, Chicago: Gateway.

Nesbit W. 1995. Is Killing No Worse Than Letting Die? *Journal of Applied Philosophy* 12(1): 101–105.

Pereira J. 2011. Legalizing euthanasia or assisted suicide: The illusion of safeguards and controls. *Current oncology* (Toronto, Ont.), 18(2): e38–e45.

Vaughn L. 2010. *Bioethics, Principles, Issues and Cases.* New York: Oxford University Press.

Vallentyne P. 2012. *Oxford Handbook of Political Philosophy.* New York: Oxford University Press.

Singer P. 2003. "Volumtary euthanasia" an utilitarian perspective. *Bioethics* 175(6): 526–541.

Court Decisions

De Rechtspraak Den Haag v. 11.09.2019—09/837356-18. Available at: https://uitspraken.rechtspraak.nl/inziendocument?id=ECLI:NL:RBDHA:2019:10:650. Accessed: 14.01.2021.

Hoge Raad v. 21. 4. 2020—19/04910. Available at: https://uitspraken.rechtspraak.nl/inziendocument?id=ECLI:NL:HR:2020: 712; https://uitspraken.rechtspraak.nl/inziendocument?id=ECLI:NL:HR. Accessed: 14.01.2021.

BVerfG, Judgment of the Second Senate of 26 February 2020—2 BvR 2347/15, paras. 1–343. Available at: http://www.bverfg.de/e/rs20200226_2bvr234715en.html. Accessed: 11.02.2021.

Yael Lavi

What is Wrong with the American Association of Suicidology Statement?

Abstract

"'Suicide' is not the same as 'physician aid in dying'" proclaims the American Association of Suicidology 2017 statement.[1] Nevertheless, I argue that (1) this pragmatic distinction is grounded in the scientific-medical approach to suicide, which focuses on parameters of objectivity and rationality that are at least questionable. (2) The weakness of the distinction suggests that the AAS statement may draw the bull's eye around the arrow, i.e. it seeks to bypass the epistemological and ethical challenge that voluntary death confronts us with by denying the rationality of the act or by doubting suicidal agency on the grounds of pathological irrationality. By doing so, (3) it fails to grasp the complex and reluctant nature of suicidal thought as an (all too) human phenomenon and may even undermine its own purpose.

Keywords: AAS, anti-logic, death, pathology, rationality, suicide

Suicide and physician aid in dying

"'Suicide' is not the same as 'physician aid in dying'" is the title of a statement published by the American Association of Suicidology (AAS) board in August 2017. The AAS, a nationally recognized NGO founded in 1968 by Edwin S. Shneidman, a clinical psychologist who largely shaped suicide dis-

[1] American Association of Suicidology, (2017). "*Suicide" Is not the Same as "Physician Aid in Dying.*" Available at: https://suicidology.org/wp-content/uploads/2019/07/AAS-PAD-Statement-Approved-10.30.17-ed-10-30-17.pdf. Accessed: 20.11.2019.

course through research methods and terms such as "psychache," "psychological autopsy," "pseudocide notes" as well as the notion of "suicidology" itself, actively promotes the prevention of suicide through research, public awareness programs, education and training (Farberow 1993, pp. 337–345; Litman et al. 1963, pp. 924–929; Shneidman 1993; Shneidman and Farberow 1957). Since its inception the AAS is actively promotes the prevention of suicide through research, public awareness programs, education and training. In response to the legalization developments of *aid in dying* in a number of jurisdictions,[2] the AAS released the above statement, which was formulated as a two-phase model convened and consolidated by Margaret Battin, one of the leading bioethics researchers in the field of end-of-life issues and suicide in particular.

Based on 15 points of difference, and a short acknowledgment regarding "the possibility of overlap between suicide and physician aid in dying" (AAS 2017, p. 4), the AAS's statement concludes with the following: "the practice of physician aid in dying, also called "physician assisted suicide," "Death with Dignity," and "medical aid in dying," is distinct from the behavior that has been traditionally and ordinarily described as "suicide"... Such deaths (i.e., physician-assisted deaths, or physician aid-in-dying (PAD)) should not be considered as cases of suicide, and are therefore a matter outside the central focus of the AAS" (AAS 2017, p. 4). Likewise, it asserts that "'physician-assisted suicide' in itself constitutes a critical reason why these distinct death categories are so often conflated, and should be deleted from use" (AAS 2017, p. 4). Although not made explicit in the document itself, as Battin herself admits, the policy implications seem to be that (1) "the suicide prevention clinician or worker does not have a professional obligation to try to prevent clear, legal cases of aid in dying" and that (2) "in such cases there would be no professional objection to serve as an advisor or to provide a mental status assessment of the patient who requests aid in dying" (Battin 2019, p. 776), as may be required by the US laws.

The contrast between suicide and PAD, it must be admitted, is rather "old news," as it has been discussed over the last four decades as part of the *right to die* debate. With the deliberate political purpose of destigmatizing assisted dying, advocates of the *right to die* approach have dissociated their cause from "suicide" and its popular connotations. By using scientific "value-neutral" terms, and speaking of choice, options, compassion and dignity,[3] this anti-suicide but pro-assisted dying discourse is constructed in such a way

[2] As of this writing, in some form or variation, PAD is legally available in eleven US states, Canada, Germany, Belgium, Switzerland, Luxembourg, the Netherlands, Colombia, and at least part or all of Australia.

[3] See for instance: Death with Dignity. *Terminology of Assisted Dying*. Available at: https://www.deathwithdignity.org/terminology/. Accessed: 02.10.2010.

that, as Michael Cholbi demonstrates, does not assert a "right to die" (roughly speaking: the *right to die* is the freedom from legal interference in bringing about one's own death, either on one's own or with the assistance of others), but rather a *right to certain modes of dying* (Cholbi 2019, p. 1).[4] Nevertheless, the AAS statement is still quite exceptional against this background, most obviously because it does not explicitly speak for or against the legalization of PAD and, more implicitly, because it does not contain any moral claim for example about the "sanctity" or "value of life"—nor does it address the common discourse of rights: liberty, dignity, property, autonomy, etc.

In fact, the absence of the latter, i.e., the concept of *autonomy*, from the statement is rather puzzling given that the only noticeable difference between suicide and PAD lies in the active involvement of an "other" (namely a family member, legal representative, or health professional) in the process. This difference, however, carries considerable ethical implications for the "other," more than for the one who wishes to die. In this respect, while the moral import of suicide (i.e. "self-killing") may be contingent, "killing someone who is not me" (or assisting in her/his death) is undoubtedly a moral issue. Put differently: while suicide may *not* be a moral issue, if help is required to carry it out, it obviously becomes one. Thus, in contrast to cases where no reason or explanation is needed (when one kill oneself in a manner that makes no moral claim on the other) in cases of assisted suicide the cooperation of the "other" is needed and conditioned by explanation based reasoned consent. In this respect, the rejection of the conceptual similarity between suicide and PAD plays an integral role for the AAS, as I hope to show.

Basically, the AAS's stance can be summarized as follows: while PAD may be an optimal solution to control the circumstances of the end of one's life's end by alleviating the inevitable suffering expected at the final stages of an incurable illness, which may be rationally and objectively justified on medical, moral, and cultural grounds by the patient, his/her relatives, and society as a whole, suicide is wrong, because it contradicts all of the above. But is this so? And, to be more specific, are the criteria of rationality and objectivity so unequivocal in that case? As space is limited here, I cannot delve into refuting or rejecting each and every one of the statement's 15 "points of difference." Instead, I will briefly touch on two plausible, seemingly contradictory (perhaps complementary) lines of argumentation: on the one hand, I will object to the "irrationality premise" (here I will largely follow Cholbi's 2019 argument); on the other hand, following Jean Améry (1999) and others, I will argue that the phenomenon of voluntary death should not and cannot be discussed in terms

---

4 I owe special thanks to Michael Cholbi for his willingness to let me read and quote from his unpublished conference paper. Cf. Cholbi 2019.

of rationality and objectivity and, hence, the application of these standards is at least problematic if not a categorical mistake.

Nonetheless, before digging into the task, a preliminary note is required regarding the definition of suicide, or rather, its absence. For there is no consensus regarding the definition of suicide, its essential features, or the exact limits of its phenomenal scope. As the riddle is not accidental, (although the full argument is beyond the scope this paper) embracing Peter Windt's *"open-textured" concept of suicide* will suffice. Windt's conceptualization "deny that there is some nuclear set of characteristics which is to be found in all cases of suicide—some core, indispensable characteristics—and in no other cases" (1980, p. 40). Accordingly, using the Wittgensteinian notion of *family resemblance*, the sharp boundary drawn by the AAS between suicide and PAD dissolves. All the more so when focus on voluntary death phenomena from the first-person perspective. Respectively, statement's points no. 10, 11, 12, and 14 will remain beyond the scope of my argument, as it addresses 2nd & 3rd person's considerations which derived from a particular contingent (mis)conception.[5]

Autonomy, death with dignity and time

Now, let's take for example the statement's first point of difference no. 1:[6]

> Under US law, the patient requesting aid in dying must be diagnosed by two independent physicians as terminally ill, defined as death expected within six months. In suicide, a life that could have continued indefinitely is cut short. PAD is not a matter of life or death; it is a matter of a foreseeable death occurring a little sooner but in an easier way, in accord with the patient's wishes and values, vs. death later in a potentially more painful and protracted manner (AAS 2017, p. 2).

According to the AAS, allegedly, in cases of PAD, the choice in question involves "one form of death over another," not "death over life." This implies that suicidal ideation introduces death into a state of affairs in which it did not previously exist, whereas the terminally ill are immersed in a situation where the harm of death have been already forced by the illness, so all that is left is to ensure a "good death" by managing the process. However the pos-

[5] Point #10 refers to the differences in legal status and consequences of the two acts. Point #11: refers to the "the impact on bereavement in family members." Point #12: refers to the "substantial social stigma"; "a considerable burden for bereaved families or other persons involved." Point #14: Point #12: refers to the "forensic and other costs" ; "dilemmas of publicity"(AAS 2017, pp. 3–4).

[6] More references in the AAS statement to the rationality of the act (see points no. 2, 5, 7, 9, and 15) are also vulnerable to this kind of argument.

sibility of dying exists in all human lives from the moment of born, whether we acknowledge it or not. Sometimes death's time is predictable and sometimes not. Sometimes it is possible to postpone death, Sometimes not. In this sense, everyone is "the individual who is already facing death" (cf. point no. 3), hence six months of life are still an amount of life, even a meaningful amount as been suggested along the AAS statement. Therefore, shortening it, **is** a matter of "life or death" all things considered.

Suicide, contend the AAS, reflects "misperception" of the "desperate" and "impulsive" person who wishes to die (cf. point no. 2). As opposed to other cases of intentional self-inflicted death that are branded as altruistic and heroic, this notion of "depressed" or "nihilistic" suicide as it known in literature, is often characterized in terms of irrationality.[7] In PAD argues the AAS, death is chosen by those who wants desperately to live (AAS 2017, p. 2) but given the circumstances, wish to avoid unnecessary pain and loss of autonomy by choosing the option of death (similarly to the altruistic/heroic self-inflicted death justifications).

Cholbi's argument clarifies, this semantic and rhetorical shift is misguided not only because it reduces the question of human liberty to determining whether *life is or isn't worth living*, to the issue of control over one's death, but because it rests on a false contrast between "choosing to die" and "choosing the circumstances of one's death."

On a purely logical level, "choosing death for the sake of being dead" does not seem to be a coherent and practical goal, as death is not a state of being. My death exceeds any my lives-experience and therefore exceeds representation or intentionality. As Epicurus asserted, "[d]eath is nothing to us, since when we are, death has not come, and when death has come, we are not" or, as Wittgenstein put it: "death is not an event in life: we do not live to experience death" (1922, § 6.4311, p. 88). Thus, as Devine demonstrated long ago, rational decision, which is by definition a teleological calculation in essence, seems to be incompatible with death as Devine demonstrated long ago (Devine 1978, pp. 23–31). Furthermore, as all humans are mortal, to take self inflicted death action *as* an act of "choosing death" seems senseless, because no one can choose not to die. We are all compelled by death whether we like it or not.

The real meaning of the intentional act toward self inflicted death, is not whether or not to die, but rather *if and how one exercises agency with respect to one's certain death*, primarily by choosing the timing and the means, based on her values, judgment, and capabilities. On this account there is no sense in seeks to differentiate between PAD and suicide based on the degree of

[7] A soldier who jumps on a grenade to save his comrades, a man who set himself on fire in protest of injustice, King Saul who falls on his sword so as not to fall captive or Socrates who drinks the cup of poison, and so on.

"the act rationality,"[8] as both PAD and suicide acts are not about "wishing for" death for its own sake but accepting the risk of dying as a means to one's desired end. It follows that if one responds positively to the *if*, then the justifications for the different variations of *how* and *when* is derives from the same ethical and logical starting point for both suicide and PAD. In this regard, justification of the terminality criterion (i.e., death expected within six months), which underlies the distinction between suicide and PAD, may be questionable: ***If*** PAD is, indeed, limited to the terminally ill, what does **terminal** mean in practice? Not only that the reliability of those death prognoses tends to be quite poor, but one should bear in mind that the PAD's six months prognosis standard, was retrieved from the hospice qualifications standards, which seems to rest **no less** on institutional financial issues than on medical consideration. It then seems plausible, that the time restriction is valid only if it is understood as a type of evidence or "index of suffering" by which it can be estimated that one's current or future suffering makes one's hastened death an advantage. But, if six months of potential suffering is the determining factor that grants the right to die, why suffer for years or decades with an incurable and untreatable illness such as in cases of chronic pain or mental pain? Let us push this line of argument a little further, as Battin herself often does (Battin 1991, pp.73–80; Battin 1994; Battin and Kious 2019, pp. 29–39). If suffering, autonomy, and dignity are the criteria by which the right to die is determined, why should it be limited to medical conditions alone?[9]

Rational or irrational choice?

The AAS's answer to this question may concealed in the statement's point no. 2;

> The person with a terminal illness does not necessarily want to die [...] Suicide, by contrast [...] typically stems from unrelenting psychological pain and despair (AAS 2017, p. 2).

This false contrast between a claim regarding the motivation's presence and its`s direction and a claim regarding the motivation's origin or cause, hides an implicit premise about the pathological nature of suicide. In light of the AAS's second "possibility of overlap" that presumption become more explicit. According to the statement, some requests for PAD made by people with

---

[8] Roughly speaking the "rationality of the act" is usually conditioned by four criteria: the act must not bring harm to the one who wishes to die; the act is in one's own interest; the act is permissible only in hopeless conditions; and the act must be considered in light of its impact on its environment (Battin 1996, pp.114–129; Cholbi 2011, pp. 88–96; Kulp 2014).

[9] Note that in the Netherlands and Belgium for example, proof of unbearable and incurable mental suffering is a legal ground for euthanasia.

terminal illnesses may be closer to conventional suicides in character where traditional treatment for depression "may well play a role," request that frequently fail to satisfy PAD requirements (AAS 2017, p. 4). That is to say, the terminally ill (or chronic pain) patient's decision to die, is objectively justified and rational because her suffering is unbearable and incurable, while the so-called "depressed" person's decision to die is objectively irrational, and therefore unjustified, as her suffering is not unbearable nor incurable.[10]

Both public and the state places the authority to judge whether a person is rational or not in the hands of the health system, first and foremost by psychiatrists and psychologists, which tends to the link between rationality, "suicidal ideation" and mental illness pathologies. While persuasive philosophical arguments in favor of rationally chosen suicide have been made in the past, even by Battin herself (1991, 1994, 1996, 2019), the AAS statement still relies heavily on the axiom of causal relationship between suicide, pathology and irrationality. That approach appears in almost half of the statement's points of difference (see points no. 2, 3, 6, 7, 8, 9, and 13), either implicitly— in concepts such as "impulsivity" and "tunnel vision" (AAS 2017, p. 2); "unrelenting psychological pain" and "sense of isolation" as well as the inability to objectively assess a situation (AAS 2017, pp. 2–3)—or more explicitly such as in point no. 8:

> Suicide [...] is much more common among those with mental illness, where it may be a complex byproduct influenced by anhedonia, impaired thinking, cognitive distortion and constriction, impaired problem-solving, anxiety, perseveration, agitation, personality disorders, and/or helplessness and hopelessness (AAS 2017, p. 3).

In other words, suicidology understands the very judgment that rejects life as unworthy, i.e. the "depressed" suicidal thought, as an indication of mental pathology (psychological, biological, or cognitive failure, etc.), while mental pathology indicates a deficiency in reasoning. That is, it delineate the suicidal thought itself as irrational by definition. Nonetheless, this tautology raises the worry that the scientific hypothesis of suicidology may be based on circular reasoning and subject to a "compulsory ontology of pathology" to use Ian Marsh's (2010) words.

It should first be noted that, according to recent studies, terminally ill patients and people suffering from incurable pain are disproportionately susceptible to depression and anxiety, that 25–75% of terminally ill patients suffer from depression, anxiety, or both, and that mental suffering plays a much more crucial role in the desire to die than the intensity of pain (Asghar-Ali et al. 2013, pp. 926–933; Block 2000, pp. 209–218; Calandre et al. 2011,

---

[10] The "rationality of the person" conditioned in the literature by five criteria: the ability to reason; the presence of a realistic worldview; the possession of adequate information; a low degree of ambivalence; and a free decision-making process (Battin 1996; Cholbi 2011; Kulp 2014).

pp. 1889–1893; Calandre et al. 2018, pp. 537–548; Fine 2001, pp. 130–133, Mystakidou et al. 2005, pp. 258–262; Tang and Crane 2006, pp. 575–586; Wilson et al. 2007, pp. 314–323; Wolfe et al. 2011, pp. 94–101).[11] So it might be reasonable to question the AAS's artificial distinction between the terminal patient's desire to die and that of the depressed suicidal person. Accordingly, the alleged distinction between suffer that stems from depression or is simply due to highly distressing life events, to that caused by terminal illness overlooks the fact that debilitating human issues are not necessarily medical in nature (cf. Baechler 1979, p. 11). That is to say, preferring death to a life of suffering, disgrace, and anguish is to view death as the best option under realistic conditions, and as such as a rational choice "even if," as Cholbi emphasizes, "it would not be the best option under counterfactual conditions" (2019, p. 7).

Moreover, and without underestimating the productive and valuable contributions of established quantitative research efforts, there is "no indisputable evidence for the claim that suicide always, or almost always is a consequence of mental disorder" (Hjelmeland and Knizek 2017, p. 489). Indeed a growing number of voices have recently pointed out that the field of suicidology has become too narrowly focused on questions of individual mental deficits, as well as too wedded to positivist research methodologies, and thus tends to exclude from consideration facts, methods, evidence, insights and interpretations that do not fit well with these models (White et al. 2016, p. 2). As Marsh and Hjelmeland among others indicate, there is plausible reason to suspect the validity of some of the empirical evidence due to built-in methodological distortions and biases, some of which may stem from common features of scientific practice itself, such as psychological autopsies.[12] Other biases, rooted in historical, moral and religious traditions, norms and values, valid or not as the case may be, implicitly underlie the premises and goals of medico-scientific inquiry. As modern secular liberal society turns to science in search of a unifying explanatory principle that could validate values. Thus, what was once a sin against God, or a crime against the sovereign (first the slave owner, then the feudal lord and finally the state), then became pathological.

[11] In addition, studies also show that, more than the current degree of suffering, it is the anticipation of the imminent return of intense suffering that plays a crucial role in the desire to die (Sullivan 2005, pp. 256–257).

[12] The methodological problem with PA may appear as a result of data that is based on second- and third-hand reporting, although a large number of the questions deal with feelings and emotions that can only be reliably reported first-hand, or of data that has been collected from small sample groups, usually family members of the suicidal person, who may not necessarily be fully aware of his or her feelings, thoughts and experiences. Likewise, a psychopathological bias may appear in quantitative research due to the wording of the questions (in qualitative studies where the interviewees were not specifically asked about mental illnesses, the incidence of mental pathology was much lower) or to both researchers and interviewees sharing the very prevalent, commonsense perception of suicide as a mental illness (Hjelmeland et al. 2012, pp. 605–626).

The invention of "suicidality" (i.e., the grouping of various phenomena—from thoughts of death ideation through self-harm to self-killing—under one clinical umbrella based on causality assumption, supposedly proven in the form of a mental disorder), has been reinforced by tremendous developments in medical research and technology that extends life expectancy and alleviates pain. Consequently, the suicidal subject (now the "patient" or "research object") becomes passive: if suicide is a symptom of illness rather than the result of rational judgment, it is not freely chosen but forced on the suicidal person, such that his/her autonomy is reduced and the power over his/her life is relinquished to external parties: family, psychiatrists, and state authorities. Neurologists and geneticists focus on biological pathology, while psychiatrists and psychologists focus on mental or cognitive pathology, writing prescriptions for antidepressants and referring patients to welfare services for treatment. Yet, the assumption that "healing from suicide" is possible by reducing mental pain through psychotherapy or neurochemical balancing, might be questionable. In this manner it is important to consider three reservations: 1) It is not certain that the eradication of mental pain is always possible. 2) The side effects of the treatment may be too high a price to pay for pain eradication; thus, it is not always desirable. 3) Clinical efforts are directed more at changing the subject's inner (mental/cognitive) rather than external conditions, which may be the real cause of his/her distress.

Additionally, focusing on the patient's psychopathological profile ignores the power that political, historical, social, cultural, or gender norms hold over the individual, that may cause *anomie* conditions (Durkheim 2002) and distress and in the first place. The fact that suicidal ideation may result from despair, helplessness, hopelessness, isolation, and loneliness, is not in dispute here. But the identification of these elements as pathological seems unfounded, even wrong, as it fails to grasp the complexity of the (all too) human phenomenon of broken trust in the world: in social reality, in mutual responsibility, and in one's ability to manifest one's subjectivity.

Lastly, it is worth remarking that even from a practical point of view there might be an inherent shortcoming in the preventive strategy promoted by the AAS to "heal" the suicidal individual and bring him/her back into the non-suicidal human community.[13] As Kulp (2014, p.121) stresses, suicidology "look implicitly or explicitly to promote and protect the interests of the society of people who are not suicidal." Again, without diminishing the merits of medical and psychological treatment, to deny the fact that their notion of "recovery" is strongly involves with "the acceptance of cognitive values which are based on an affirmative stance" (Clements 1980, p. 105) and thereby confirms the suicidal person's sense of misfit and alienated, would be naive.

---

[13] Available at: https://suicidology.org/about. Accessed: 20.11.2019.

Beyond the logic of life?

A different line of argument in opposition to the AAS statement asserts that rationality and objectivity have essentially nothing to do with suicide. Both science and morality attempt to define voluntary death based on a systematic, coherent and general system, explained and managed by the categorization of "right" and "wrong." Yet, this judgmental framework may be wrong in regard to suicide, either because of the problematic nature of concepts such as "rationality," "objectivity," and "autonomy" and their prevalent neoliberal medical significance or because, in its essence and radical singularity, voluntary death rejects reasoning and justification. In this regard, to claim that suicide is rational (or irrational) could be tantamount to claiming that the number five is red (or green).

The former critique, which comes mainly from postmodern, postcolonial and feminist thought, as vast as it is diverse, offers both ontological and epistemological considerations that should be addressed seriously. Roughly speaking this critique rejects the atomistic ontological presupposition that identifies the fully-developed self as a rational self-sufficient single autonomous. In doing so, it opens the door to a more non-hierarchical, organic view and interdependent relational paradigm, at all levels of social, scientific and political structures. Epistemologically, it acknowledges first and foremost that every approach has a certain starting point, a non-objective, subjectively grounded perspective rooted in the experience of lived embodiment. Thus, a different kind of research question may appear for the nature of science itself is in question. A question that to use Donna Haraway's words:

> [...] is about objectivity as positioned rationality. Its images are not the products of escape and transcendence of limits (the view from above) but the joining of partial views and halting voices into a collective subject position that promises a vision of the means of ongoing finite embodiment, of living within limits and contradictions—of views from somewhere (Haraway 1988, p. 590).

For the sake of brevity, I will not develop this line of thought here, however it is worth keeping it in mind as we address the latter critique, i.e. that applying terms of rationality and objectivity to suicide is a categorical mistake. I will try to explain this stance using Jean Améry's (1976/1999) distinction between the "logic of life" and the "anti-logic of death." (In this respect, it may be useful to mention its roots in Sartrean philosophy, mainly the concept of embodied consciousness, which manifests its subjectivity by projecting itself into the world through constant, pre-reflective acts of negation. As such, not only is the human condition dominated by the a-rationality of any particular project, but it can never be fully mediated, rationalized or defined due to the contingent, particular and singular nature of *le vécu*, the "lived experience").

According to Améry, the *logic of life*, or the "logic of being," means that "all logical conclusions that we draw in statements about life are constantly bound to the fact of this life" (Améry 1976/1999, p. 18). Améry's *logic of life* is based on an unmediated ontological notion of being in the world that stimulate a pre-reflective epistemological framework, which in turn enables the establishment of (implicit or explicit) mutual knowledge, relations, abstractions, and norms. As such, the logic of life may be captured by the equation, Body = Sensation = Life, to paraphrase Améry's well-known equation, "Body = Pain = Death," taken from his memoir, "Torture" (Améry 1980, pp. 33–34; Lavi 2019, pp. 261–284). The feasibility of both equations confirms that, despite the fact that the logic of life is forced upon us with almost exclusive power until our last breath, in some cases it is violated so one finds oneself painfully oscillating between the *logic of life* and the *anti-logic of death*. In contrast to being, death is not an object of human experience. Death cannot be bound to any categories of being through which human perception and consciousness understand the world. It cannot bear any content for human intentionality; therefore, any representation of death will be representation of an absences (Critchley 2004, p. 16). The applicability range of this absence, I argue, applies for Améry's *anti-logic of death*: not only as *absence of life* kind of recognition, but the *absence in life*, evident in the paradoxical resonance of death (the absolute nothingness) within human reality.

To borrow the analogy of a black hole for a moment, the anti-logic of death is actually the gravitational field of death, which in itself lies behind the event-horizon. It is an absence that quite often cannot be subordinated to explanation or reasoning, but only recognized by negation: despair as an absence of hope, illness as an absence of health, contempt and worthlessness as an absence of dignity and finally the absence of habitual faith, or to put it better *a loss of trust in the world*. The existential loss of trust (not an a priori lack of trust, but rather the loss of it) has an epistemological, physical, and emotional aspects. To acknowledge the absence is to endorse anti-logic of death. This experience may inflict an enduring sense of alienation that revolts against the *logos* itself (and also vice versa), undermining the sufficiency of reason and the adequacy of proportion, opinion, expectation and pleas, by rejecting basic classifications such as "true" or "false" as "categories of being." The intrinsic bias toward life and it's "naive realism" mechanism are challenged by this fundamentally different structure of intentionality toward the world that produces different style of hope, much limited in its scope and its potential contents (Ratcliffe 2013, p. 16).[14] From this point of view, the seemingly necessary link between facts and values on which the logic of life

[14] It should be noticed that Ratcliffe refers to traumatic experience, however, the criterion for "trauma" are not unequivocal so it can be as broad as it can be narrow and limited. I apply it here in its broad sense, nonetheless, a further exploration of this issue is required.

is based is no longer mandatory, so life itself becomes a contingent matter which could never be converge under general and necessary *a priori* justification or reasoning.

The shock waves of the anti-logic of death reach to the shores the logic of life; unveils its fragility and absurd nature: it acknowledges existential loneliness and dependency as well as the unmet human need for meaning; it admits that in its essence, trust is conditioned by uncertainty and vulnerability but also admits that without this unjustifiable trust, life is neither desirable nor possible. Granted, this is an outrage from the *logic of life's* point of view, which, I remind you, is prescribed for human beings until their last breath.

In this paradoxical state of affairs, it seems that rational justification is futile as well as nonsensical from the standpoint of the suicidal person, and as such an inappropriate consideration. It is nonsense not only because of the enigmatic nature of death but rather, and more importantly, because the concepts used to describe a life subject to the *anti-logic of death* are utterly foreign to those who exclusively subscribe to the *logic of life*, logic that judge cognitive values based on an affirmative stance. This gap between the two stances is pre-reflective, and it affects the agent's relation to rationality and therefore as Clements suggested: "In a real sense, an individual who does not value existence does not value anything at all, and to apply tools of cognitive values to this primary affect is to deny him his validity in a totally arbitrary fashion" (Clements 1980, p. 107).

Conclusions

So, what's wrong with the AAS statement? Well, to put it briefly: it draws the bull's eye around the arrow. A longer answer is that, philosophically, the distinction between suicide and PAD may prove to be unsound and unjustified, as it overlooks the fundamental existential question (i.e., "to be or not to be") posed in both cases. However, in terms of *use*, i.e., in order to support the everyday valuable merits of the AAS, this distinction is essential. If the "depressed suicide" and PAD are privet cases of suicide (and they are), then they belong to the same conceptual and moral category, so that the considerations in favor of the latter are equally valid for the former. But, if this is the case, on what grounds can the AAS justify its mission to prevent suicide?

The moral premise, or should I say the "moral sentiment," on which suicidology bases its scientific justifications rests on value judgments that identify "life as the highest good" and promote the "sanctity of life," "the duty to prevent unnecessary death" (Leenaars 2010, p. 17). Nonetheless, these value judgments regarding suicide are not unbiased, nor can be justified *a priori* (at least not outside of a religious framework), and they certainly cannot be subject to any empirical, objective justification that has a general and necessary application. My argument is inspired by G.E.M. Anscombe's critique in "Modern Moral Philosophy" (Anscombe 1958), which is mainly directed at the reliance on religious concepts in a secular framework: that is to say, when religious tradition has been rejected and divine sovereignty eliminated, the concepts of "ought," "evil," "permissible" and so on are no more than empty words. To be sure, Anscombe does not reject all talk about moral obligation but rather frames it as part of human practice or, to put it differently, of understanding other people's means to know what they are taking on themselves to be and how they understand their acts (Anscombe 1958, pp. 1–19).

It seems that the scientific approach, which focuses on parameters of objectivity and rationality, is supposed to bypass the existential dilemma (i.e. "to be or not to be") as well as the moral dilemma (i.e. the permissibility of suicide and of assisted suicide) by simply denying the rationality of the act or questioning the agency of suicidal individuals on grounds of pathological irrationality. In both cases, paternalistic intervention can be justified. But it is not. Hence, a similarity between suicide and PAD has intolerable moral and political implications: for, by sanctioning one voluntary death while prohibiting another, the AAS in effect "plays God." To be honest, it is not only an abstract philosophical dilemma but also a very concrete and practical one, that expose the AAS to criminal and civil accusations as well as insurance claims. And, no, this is not a cynical critique.

Voluntary death presents a significant epistemological, ethical and political challenge. In undermining the structure of reasoning and behavioral habits, suicide denounces "the rules of the game". It reopens old wounds such as "truth," "justice," "good," and "freedom," which may continue to bleed, for the singular, complex and absurd nature of voluntary death, emphasized by the seemingly contradictory, yet actually complementary objections presented here, seems to leave us in aporia (ἀπορία).

Perhaps an alternative philosophical exploration that lies beyond the current bioethical and Suicidological discourse is needed, one that seeks for more adequate expressions and a more precise analysis of the situation's components as well as their modes of conceptualization. "Describing" death ideation cannot only be a matter of translating facts into words, but rather an act of attention and imagination, an inquiry that is "engaged in shaping the language of particularity" as Cora Diamond suggests (1993, pp.128–153). By committing to this kind of exploration, we might gain an alternative understanding of what it means to be mortal. This insight might not only raise additional philosophical questions but also demand different medico-scientific definitions as well as modes of therapeutic work. It also raises questions concerning the degree to and form in which society and state institution should or could be involved in a personal end of life. In other words, it is a worthy philosophical undertaking to not only explain or clarify the suicide phenomena but also to push the mind's limits by expand the boundaries of language, shaping and changing ethical reality itself. Nonetheless, and despite my great fondness for the idea expressed in Diamond's notion, according to which the "important thing then is not what answer you give, but your willingness to look, i.e., you're not laying down general philosophical conditions" (Diamond 1991, p. 21), it must be admitted that there may have some disturbing ethical and political implications when it comes to matters of life and death.

References

AAS 2017. American Association of Suicidology. 2017. *"Suicide" Is not the Same as "Physician Aid in Dying."* Available at: https://suicidology.org/wp-content/uploads/2019/07/AAS-PAD-Statement-Approved-10.30.17-ed-10-30-17.pdf. Accessed: 20.11.2019.

Améry J. 1976/1999. *On Suicide: A Discourse on Voluntary Death.* Transl. J.D. Barlow. Bloomington: Indiana UP.

Améry J. 1980. Torture. In *At the Mind's Limits: Contemplations by a Survivor on Auschwitz and Its Realities*, 21–40. Bloomington: Indiana University Press.

Anscombe G. 1958. Modern moral philosophy. *Philosophy* 33(124): 1–19. Available at: http://www.jstor.org/stable/3749051. Accessed: 10.10.2020.

Asghar-Ali A.A., Wagle K.C., Braun U.K. 2013. Depression in terminally ill patients: Dilemmas in diagnosis and treatment. *Journal of Pain and Symptom Management* 45(5): 926–933.

Baechler J. 1979. *Suicides.* Oxford: Basil Blackwell.

Battin M.P. 1991. Rational suicide: How can we respond to a request for help? *Crisis: The Journal of Crisis Intervention and Suicide Prevention* 12(2): 73–80.

Battin M.P. 1994. *The Least Worst Death: Essays in Bioethics on the End of Life.* New York: Oxford University Press.

Battin M.P. 1996. *The Death Debate: Ethical Issues in Suicide.* New Jersey: Prentice Hall.

Battin M.P. 2019. Development of the AAS statement on "suicide" and "physician aid in dying." *Suicide Life Threat Behav.* 49(3): 774–776.

Battin M.P., Kious B.M. 2019. Physician aid-in-dying and suicide prevention in psychiatry: A moral crisis? *American Journal of Bioethics* 19(10): 29–39.

Bennett, A. 2017. *Suicide century: literature and suicide from James Joyce to David Foster Wallace.* Cambridge, UK: Cambridge University Press.

Block S.D. 2000. Assessing and managing depression in the terminally ill patient. ACP-ASIM End-of-Life Care Consensus Panel. American College of Physicians—American Society of Internal Medicine. *Annals of Internal Medicine* 132(3): 209–218.

Calandre E.P., Vilchez J.S., Molina-Barea R., Tovar Garcia-Leiva J.M., Hidalgo J., Rodriguez-Lopez C.M., Rico-Villademoros F. 2011. Suicide attempts and risk of suicide in patients with fibromyalgia: A survey in Spanish patients. *Rheumatology* 50(10): 1889–1893.

Calandre E.P., Rico-Villademoros F., Slim M. 2018. Suicidal behaviors in patients with rheumatic diseases: A narrative review. *Rheumatology International* 38(4): 537–548.

Cholbi M. 2011. *Suicide: The Philosophical Dimensions.* Peterborough, Ont.–London: Broadview Press.

Cholbi M. 2017. Suicide. In *The Stanford Encyclopedia of Philosophy*, ed. E.N. Zalta. Available at: https://plato.stanford.edu/archives/fall2017/entries/suicide. Accessed: 10.10.2020.

Cholbi M. 2019. Whatever happened to the right to die? In *Voluntary Death—Interdisciplinary Approaches Workshop.* Tel-Aviv.

Clements C. 1980. The ethics of not-being: Individual options for suicide. In *Suicide: The Philosophical Issues*, eds. M.P. Battin, D.J. Mayo, 104–114. New York: St. Martin's Press.

Cowley C. 2006. Suicide is neither rational nor irrational. *Ethical Theory and Moral Practice* 9(5): 495–504.

Critchley S. 2004. *Very Little—Almost Nothing: Death, Philosophy, Literature.* London–New York: Routledge.

Devine P. 1978. *Ethics of Homicide.* Ithaca: Cornell University Press.

Diamond C. 1991. *The Realistic Spirit.* Cambridge, MA: MIT Press.

Diamond C. 1993. Martha Nussbaum and the need for novels. *Philosophical Investigations* 16(2): 128–153.

Durkheim E. 1897/2002. *Suicide: A Study in Sociology.* ProQuest eBook Central. Available at: https://ebookcentral-proquest-com.rproxy.tau.ac.il/lib/tau/detail.action?docID=242097. Accessed: 10.10.2020.

Farberow N.L. 1993. Bereavement after suicide. In *Suicidology: Essays in Honor of Edwin S. Shneidman*, ed. A.A. Leenaars, 337–345. Northvale–New York–London: Jason Aronson.

Fine R.L. 2001. Depression, anxiety, and delirium in the terminally ill patient. *Baylor University Medical Center Proceedings* 14(2): 130–133.

Haraway D. 1988. Situated knowledges: The science question in feminism and the privilege of partial perspective. *Feminist Studies* 14(3): 575–599.

Hjelmeland H., Dieserud G., Dyregrov K., Knizek B.L., Leenaars A.A. 2012. Psychological autopsy studies as diagnostic tools: Are they methodologically flawed? *Death Studies* 36(7): 605–626.

Hjelmeland H., Knizek B.L. 2017. Suicide and mental disorders: A discourse of politics, power, and vested interests. *Death Studies* 41(8): 481–492.

Kulp M.J. 2014. *The Limits of Rationality: Suicidality, Affectivity, and the Rational.* PhD thesis. Loyola University Chicago. ProQuest Dissertations Publishing. Available at: http://search.proquest.com/docview/1655002275. Accessed: 22.05.2016.

Lavi Y. 2019. Between the Logic of Life and the Anti-logic of Death: Reflections on Suicidality in the Wake of Jean Améry. In *Jean Améry*, eds. Y. Ataria, A. Kravitz, E. Pitcovski, 261–284. London: Palgrave Macmillan.

Leenaars, A.A. 2010. Edwin S. Shneidman on suicide: Review. *Suicidology Online* 1: 5–18.

Litman R.E., Curphey T.J., Shneidman E.S., Farberow N.L., Tabachnick N.D. 1963. Investigations of equivocal suicides. *Journal of the American Medical Association* 184(12): 924–929.

Marsh I. 2010. *Suicide: Foucault, history and truth*. Cambridge: Cambridge University Press.

Mystakidou K., Rosenfeld B., Parpa E., Katsouda E., Tsilika E., Galanos A., Vlahos L. 2005. Desire for death near the end of life: The role of depression, anxiety, and pain. *General Hospital Psychology* 27(4): 258–262.

Ratcliffe M. 2013. What is it to lose hope? *Phenomenology and the Cognitive Sciences* 12: 597–614.

Shneidman E.S., Farberow N.L. 1957. Some comparisons between genuine and simulated suicide notes. *Journal of General Psychology* 56: 251–256.

Shneidman E.S. 1993. *Suicide as Psychache: A Clinical Approach to Self-Destructive Behavior*. Northvale–New York–London: Jason Aronson.

Stolorow R.D. 2007. *Trauma and Human Existence: Autobiographical, Psychoanalytic and Philosophical Reflections*. New York: Routledge.

Sullivan M.D. 2005. The desire for death arises from an intolerable future rather than an intolerable present. *General Hospital Psychiatry* 27(4): 256–257.

Tang N.K.Y., Crane C. 2006. Suicidality in chronic pain: A review of the prevalence, risk factors and psychological links. *Psychological Medicine* 36(5): 575–586.

Tatz C. 2001. Aboriginal suicide is different: A portrait of life and self-destruction. *Current Issues in Criminal Justice* 14(1): 127–128.

Webb D. 2010. *Thinking about Suicide: Contemplating and Comprehending the Urge to Die*. Ross-on-Wye, Herefordshire, UK: PCCS BOOKS.

White J., Marsh I., Kral M.J., Morris J. (eds.) 2016. *Critical Suicidology: Transforming Suicide Research and Prevention for the 21st Century*. Vancouver, Canada: UBC Press.

Wilson K.G., Chochinov H.M., McPherson C.J., Skirko M.G., Allard P., Chary S., Gagnon P.R., Macmillan K., De Luca M., O'Shea F., Kuhl D., Fainsinger R.L., Karam A.M., Clinch J.J. 2007. Desire for euthanasia or physician-assisted suicide in palliative cancer care. *Health Psychology* 26(3): 314–323.

Windt P. 1980. The concepts of suicide. In *Suicide: The Philosophical Issues*, eds. M.P. Battin and D.J. Mayo, 39–47. New York: St. Martin's Press.

Wittgenstein L. 1922. *Tractatus logico-philosophicus*. Transl. C.K. Ogden. London–New York: Kegan Paul, Trench, Trubner, & Co.–Harcourt, Brace & Company, Inc.

Wolfe F., Hassett A.L., Walitt B., Michaud K. 2011. Mortality in fibromyalgia: A study of 8,186 patients over thirty-five years. *Arthritis Care and Research* 63(1): 94–101.

Patrycja Zurzycka

Advance Care Planning: Health Care Agent

Abstract

Advance care planning enables patients to express *pro futuro* their autonomy and to make decisions about their therapeutic and care processes. It is the basis for the provision of holistic and individualized care. A process of dialogue between the patient and their loved ones, and health care professionals and others involved in their care, with the aim of establishing achievable goals of care consistent with the patient's preferences. One form of advance care planning is the appointment of a health care agent to make decisions on behalf of the incompetent patient based on the patient's previously expressed wishes and preferences. Therefore, it is important to appoint people close to patients who are familiar with their preferences, beliefs, and values to serve as their agent. The scope of the health care agent includes making decisions related to the therapeutic process and care to the extent to which the patient would be entitled and his health condition would allow the current expression of consent.

The institution of health care agent still does not function in the Polish legal system or the healthcare system. This situation has not been changed by Recommendation No. 11 of the Council of Europe of 2009, nor by the initiatives of the medical and legal community to create guidelines and regulate the legal basis for health care agents.

Keywords: ACP, care, patients, autonomy, health care, healthcare system

Introduction

Obtaining the patient's consent for the performance of services proposed to him is the basis of modern medical practice. The patients' will constitute the limit of medical intervention admissibility and their autonomy prevails over objective assessment of legitimacy of the actions taken. The progress of medicine has led to the emergence of new therapeutic possibilities, which often raise questions about the limits of the medical staff's duty to respect the patient's wishes and provide the best care.

As the world's demographics change (aging populations) and medical science advances, caring for adult patients with chronic illnesses who lack decision-making capacity will increasingly become an integral part of medical practice (McMahan et al. 2013; Montanari 2020; Potter and Lee 2020; Sussman et al. 2017). For these individuals, it is necessary to make decisions based on grounds other than their informed consent. One possibility is to refer to decisions made by them when they were competent to formulate them—decisions expressed autonomously *pro futuro* (Luck et al. 2017; Montanari 2020).

The concept of advance care planning (ACP) began in the 1960s and 1970s in the United States. Its introduction was associated with the recognition of each citizen's right to consent or refuse to medical services proposed, as well as the right to request the cessation of already ongoing treatment. A key moment for the development of the idea of advance care planning was the adoption of legislation in the US in 1990, which allowed patients to express *pro futuro* decisions about the treatment and therapeutic management provided to them (Brown 2003; Quenot et al. 2017). Nowadays, the possibility of advance care planning is increasingly common and operates in many healthcare systems around the world (Cheng et al. 2020; Korfage and Fried 2020; Szeroczyńska et al. 2016a). The concept of advance care planning is based on respecting patients' values, goals, and preferences in the context of medical care (Sudore et al. 2010; Sudore et al. 2017a). This is possible through the promotion of patients' rights, among which respect for dignity, access to health information and the ability to express their autonomy through informed decision-making (informed consent) regarding the therapeutic and care management provided are considered the most fundamental (Aasmul et al. 2018; Hamilton 2017).

Advance care planning is recognized as a process aimed at determining the patient's preferences regarding the actions that should be taken towards him when his health condition will prevent ongoing communication and decision-making. Planning is based on effective communication between the patients, their loved ones, agents appointed to make decisions, and medical staff and others involved in the provision of care (Grądalski and Kochan 2017; Sudore et al. 2017a; Sussman et al. 2017). It most often takes the form of a discussion in which the patient is encouraged to identify and discuss his values, beliefs, and life goals in the context of health care that he wishes to receive in the future. In addition to making their own reflections, the patient's role is to engage in conversation with their family and treatment team, and to share with own preferences. Thus, advance care planning is a dynamic process that evolves with time, changes in health status (disease progression), or changes in preferences, involving the patient and all those involved in the care (both the patient's loved ones and the medical staff) (Michael et al. 2017; Quenot et al. 2017; Sussman et al. 2017). The primary role of advance care planning is to clarify the goals of future care and to help the patient's loved ones and staff make decisions in situations where the patient will not be able to communicate and establish them independently (Dunlay et al. 2016; Michael et al. 2017; Sinclair et al. 2017). Preferences for future care by the patient may be general and relate to values and life goals or existential issues. They can also be more precise and address specific situations related to hospitalization, life-sustaining treatment, or comfort and palliative care management (Grądalski and Kochan 2017; Mullick et al. 2013; Rietjens et al. 2017).

The benefits of advance care planning mainly include its provision in accordance with patient-relevant goals and values, but it also affects patients' better quality of life and reduces the frequency of persistent and aggressive therapy. In addition, it improves communication and trust between the patient and their loved ones and medical staff. It is also helpful in alleviating negative emotions, both of patients and their loved ones, related to the inevitability of the patient's deteriorating health (Carr and Luth 2019; Dunlay and Strand 2016; Grądalski et al. 2017; Hamilton 2017; Lum et al. 2018). For those receiving institutional care (nursing homes, assisted living facilities), it reduces the frequency of their hospitalizations (Michael et al. 2017), and for terminally ill patients, it increases the desire for hospice care (Grądalski et al. 2017; Hamilton 2017) and reduces anxiety for patients as well as their loved ones (Lum et al. 2018).

Advance care planning should not be a one-time event but a reflection that continues throughout a person's adult life. Such reflections on values and life goals should be undertaken in the context of broadly defined human well-being, the accepted concept of health and illness, but also the realities of primary or specialist medical care (Potter and Lee 2020; Prince-Paul and DiFranco 2017; Schellinger et al. 2018). It is advisable that discussions about advance care planning be initiated early in adulthood and address general human values in the context of medical care and also seek to identify a person who could potentially perform the role of health care agent. Reflections and conversations about life values and goals should be conducted especially at key points in life, such as reaching adulthood, getting married or starting a family, and the birth of offspring. As health status changes and when a serious illness is diagnosed or when functioning deteriorates in the face of an existing disorder (chronic illness), planning should be less general and more focused on specific situations, procedures, or treatment options. Such care planning allows for a thorough understanding by care planners of the importance of their role in deciding future care and therapeutic management

(Michael et al. 2017). It is advisable to periodically review the determinations made in advance care planning especially while the patient is still capable of actively participating in these conversations. Decision review should be conducted especially when there is a change in the patient's perception of quality of life, changes in values and preferences due to progressive disease, the emergence of new therapeutic options, and a change in the patient's location (e.g., transfer to institutional long-term care or hospital). Also, during the period when the patient is unable to communicate and make decisions, the agent and those involved in the care should review and revise the arrangements made in relation to the current situation (Hamilton 2017).

The final result of an advance care planning process can be various types of decisions and the attestations documenting them. A formalized example of *pro futuro* care planning are advance directives (ADs) (Prince-Paul and DiFranco 2017; Quenot et al. 2017; Sinclair et al. 2017). These can take the form of patient-drafted living will—a statement of preferred medical management—or the appointment of a health care agent to decide on the health care provided in place of the patient (Bomba 2017; Carr and Luth 2017; Dunlay and Strand 2016; Escher et al. 2014; McMahan et al. 2013; Potter and Lee 2020). Sometimes patients' only choice of care planning is to talk and verbally communicate their preferences, values, and directions for future behavior to medical staff and loved ones (Michael et al. 2017; Sinclair et al. 2017; Sudore et al. 2017b).

Advance care planning—health care agent

As mentioned above, one form of advance care planning is the appointment of a health care agent. The health care agent is a person chosen by the patient, whose task is to act on his behalf in the area of decision-making and giving consent for activities carried out within the scope of medical care provided. This applies to situations in which the patient, due to medical condition, is not able to independently exercise his autonomy and right to self-determination through ongoing decision-making and communication (Bomba 2017; Luck et al. 2017; Potter et al. 2020; Szeroczyńska et al. 2016a; Wendler 2017). The scope of authority available to a patient-designated agent overlaps with the scope that the patient would have if he were able to make and express his own preferences. However, the health care agent's decisions and actions should not be based on his subjective judgment, but should appeal to the patient's values, preferences, and previously expressed autonomous will (Boerner et al. 2013; Bomba 2017; McMahan et al. 2013; Vig et al. 2006). Family members of the patient or unrelated individuals close to the patient are usually appointed to act as the health care agent. When making this choice, most patients assume that the people closest to them best understand their preferences and thus will be the guarantor of the implementation of their wishes (Carr and Luth 2019; Kim et al. 2017; Torke et al. 2014).

In making alternative decisions, agents should first consider the guidance given to them directly by the patient. If it is not possible to make a decision based on the information at hand (e.g., in the case of a situation about which the patient has not explicitly expressed his opinion), it is advisable to resort to interpreting the patient's wishes based on his general preferences, values, and beliefs (including those related to spirituality or religion) and decisions previously made by the patient. A final option considered may be to rely on the criterion of the patient's best interests (Fritsch et al. 2013). The consensus of those involved in care as to the rightness of decisions (consensus reached within the family or among those close to the patient) and a sense of duty to the patient may also play an important role in alternative decision making (Fritsch et al. 2013; Vig et al. 2006). The support available to the health care agent and the communication between the agent and the medical staff may also influence decision making (Vig et al. 2006).

Individuals taking on the role of health care agent have varying degrees of preparation for their tasks (Kim et al. 2017; Vig et al. 2006). Alternative decision making involves the evaluation of a proposed therapeutic or care procedure and its potential benefits and burdens in relation to previously expressed patient preferences (Kim et al. 2017; Rosoff 2017). The need to focus on representing the patient's interests can lead to situations in which decisions made by the agent, although consistent with the principal's wishes, conflict with the values of a person representing the patient. There are also occasions when decisions made in accordance with the patient's preferences may not reflect what the patient's best interests would be in the agent's opinion or that of the treatment team (Detering et al. 2010; Luck et al. 2017; Vig et al. 2006; 2017; Wendler 2017). The agent may not know the patient's actual preferences or may put their own opinion above the patient's wishes (Carr and Luth 2017; Fritsch et al. 2013; Potter et al. 2020). Furthermore, agents may face difficulties in interpreting the patient's wishes in relation to specific clinical situations (i.e., way of interpreting the patient's preferences and values in the context of specific medical decisions) (Carr and Luth 2019). It is worth noting that agents are often obligated to make complex decisions regarding the management of therapy and care for their loved ones in the face of a severe and incurable disease with an unsuccessful prognosis. Having to make such difficult decisions can cause agents to experience stress, emotional tension, and anxiety related to whether they are acting appropriately for their loved ones (Kim et al. 2017; Buckley and Molina 2012; McMahan et al. 2013;

Rosoff 2017) and guilt related to the consequences of their decisions (Sulmasy et al. 2017).

Health care agent in the Polish healthcare system

The primary international norms governing *pro futuro* declarations of will and the appointment of agents are contained in a document of the Council of Europe of 2009—Recommendation of the Committee of Ministers to member states on principles concerning continuing powers of attorney and advance directives for incapacity (Council of Europe 2009). The document obliges member states to introduce solutions in healthcare systems that allow for the realization of patient autonomy *pro futuro* (in the form of permanent powers of attorney and declarations of will). According to these recommendations, the health care agent should take over the decision-making powers of the patient at the moment when he loses the actual ability to make (and communicate) his decisions. The agent is required to act in accordance with the wishes of a person being represented. Decisions made by an agent are not limited to issues related to the medical care provided but include all issues of importance to the patient. It is advisable that the power of attorney be in writing and include a description of all areas in which the agent is empowered to make decisions on behalf of the principal. The recommendation allows for the appointment of several agents who may make decisions jointly, but also act in areas specified by the person appointing them (e.g. health care agent, proxy making decisions in the area of property, etc.). Member States, in addition to introducing the above-mentioned regulations, are obliged to protect the persons appointing agents against possible abuse on their part. This protection includes the necessity to determine whether the principal's incapacity to exercise self-determination has actually occurred, to regulate issues related to appointing and registering powers of attorney, and to set the effective date of the power of attorney and the conditions under which it may be effective (Council of Europe 2009).

The current regulations in Poland do not include provisions regulating the functioning of health care agents within the meaning of the above-mentioned Recommendation (Council of Europe 2009). There are legal opinions which base the functioning of health care agents on the provisions of the Civil Code—granting a power of attorney to make decisions concerning life and health. The possibility of applying the provisions of the Civil Code is supported by the decision of the Supreme Court of April 11, 2006, which assumed that the consent for a medical procedure is a manifestation of will similar to a civil law declaration of will. According to Article 95 of the Civil Code (the concept of representation), any legal act may be performed by a representative, unless the law clearly provides otherwise (Szeroczyńska 2013). Another decision of the Supreme Court dated October 27, 2005 is also relevant—the patient's statement expressed in the case of unconsciousness, specifying the will regarding the physician's conduct in relation to the patient in treatment situations that may arise, is binding on the physician—if made in a clear and unambiguous manner (Rzecznik Praw Obywatelskich 2020).

However, both the medical authorities and some lawyers, recognize that the lack of statutory regulations in Poland on the issue of health care agent proves the impossibility of referring to this type of institution on the basis of general provisions on representation contained in the Civil Code (Pawłowski et al. 2019; Szeroczyńska 2013; Waszkiewicz 2017). The Act on the Profession of Doctor and Dentist and the Act on Patients' Rights and the Ombudsman of Patients' Rights do not indicate health care agents as entities authorized to make decisions. Alternative consent can be given by a statutory representative or a court, and in relation to the examination, also by an actual guardian (Ustawa o zawodach lekarza i lekarza dentysty, art. 32; Ustawa o prawach pacjenta i Rzeczniku praw pacjenta, art. 17) This results in situations in which, in the case of adult and incapacitated patients unable to make their own decisions, it is necessary to ask the guardianship court for permission to undertake any medical action. This applies to all situations, not just those involving increased risk (e.g., surgery). Consent must be given on a case-by-case basis for each service. It is also not possible for the court to establish a blanket consent, which is also considered invalid in the case of the patient's own consent. In everyday medical practice related to the care of patients unable to give consent, such a solution is non-functional (Szeroczyńska 2013; Waszkiewicz 2017; Rzecznik Praw Obywatelskich 2018; 2020). In practice, recourse to a court decision is rarely used, while much more often the family is asked to give consent on behalf of an incompetent patient (Grzejszczak and Szeroczyńska 2012). Another group of patients for whom the health care agent could make decisions are those who waive the right to information about their health status and thus have no basis for informed consent for the proposed medical treatment. In relation to this group of patients, the decision is not made by the court, because they do not show incapacity to make a decision, nor can it be made by a person authorized to receive information (if the patient has designated such a person) (Szeroczyńska et al. 2016a).

Due to the lack of a clearly formulated legal basis for the possibility of health care agents in Poland, attempts have been made to standardize their functioning. One of the first drafts of a law that was supposed to organize the provisions on consent and objection to treatment was a proposal made in 2013 by a group of lawyers and doctors associated with the Warsaw Hospice for Children (Projekt nowelizacji Ustawy o Prawach Pacjenta i Rzeczniku Praw Pacjenta 2013; Waszkiewicz 2017). In 2016, another effort to introduce the institution of a health care agent was made by the Polish Working Group on Ethical Issues at the End of Life. The group published its statement, in which it presented the proposals developed since 2008 for dealing with the lack of the patient's ability to make informed decisions. It also indicated the principles of appointing a health care agent, its tasks, responsibilities and implemented the solutions proposed in the Recommendation of the Council of Europe of 2009 (Szeroczyńska et al. 2016a). Support for this initiative was expressed by the Supreme Medical Council in the Statement of November 4, 2016 on the creation of an institution of health care agent in Polish law (Naczelna Rada Lekarska 2016).

The position of the Polish Working Group on Ethical Issues at the End of Life on the possibility of appointing health care proxies. The purpose of the Polish Working Group on Ethical Issues at the End of Life, established in 2008, was to develop guidelines on how to proceed in various cases related to medical decisions made with regard to persons at the end-of-life stages. This team developed a statement on the introduction and functioning of the institution of health care agent in the reality of Polish medical care (Szeroczyńska et al. 2016a; 2016b).

It was agreed that every adult person who has full legal capacity (has not been incapacitated) should have the right to appoint a health care agent to represent their interests if they lose the ability to make decisions on their own behalf or decide to waive their right to information. Also minors (above 16 years of age) should have the possibility to appoint a health care agent. However, the health care agent can make decisions only after the person appointing him has reached the age of majority (until then the legal representative decides). Any adult appointed by the patient can become a health care agent. It is important that they know the patient well so that they can make decisions in accordance with their values and beliefs. It is possible to appoint one or more people to act as health care agents (substitute health care proxies). Establishing a health care agent for only one person may raise problems in carrying out that person's functions (for example, due to lack of availability, loss of capacity to make informed decisions, or relinquishment of the agent role). In light of these potential problems, it is recommended to appoint substitute agents to take over the role of the primary agent (appointed first) in the case that the primary agent is unable (or unwilling) to perform his role. The person appointed by the patient as agent must consent to serve in this role. This consent should be in writing or verbally attested by the signatures of two witnesses (these witnesses must not have direct medical care of the patient, nor can the patient become a witness). The same rules for consent to represent the patient also apply to substitute attorneys. A power of attorney must also be made in writing and witnessed by two people (who may not be representatives of the medical team caring for the patient, the patient, non-lawyers, or people who cannot read or write) and must be dated. Powers of attorney given orally must be written by one of the witnesses. The document may be adapted to the patient's needs and abilities when it is drawn up (e.g., computer print with appropriate letter size, Braille print). Both the patient and the agent(s) must have an original copy of the power of attorney and a certification that the agent is authorized to act. For the power of attorney to be effective, it must be presented to the attending physician, who attaches copies of the power of attorney and the agent's consent to the patient's medical record. It is also advisable to create systemic solutions enabling the patient or the agent to register the power of attorney on their own in the systems that contain the patient's medical data (along with attaching electronic copies of the power of attorney and the agent's consent). The power of attorney becomes effective when the patient loses decision-making competence (both permanently and temporarily), which should be assessed by a doctor caring for the patient on medical grounds. The second situation in which a power of attorney becomes effective is when a patient waives the right to information and at the same time designates a health care agent as the person authorized to make decisions. The duration of a power of attorney depends on the patient's will, and both indefinite and time-limited forms are acceptable. The power of attorney may be revoked by the principal at any time, and the health care agent may resign from his position at any time. However, the form of revocation or resignation may be discretionary, but it is important to note this fact in the patient's medical records. In cases where the health care agent takes actions that are contrary to the patient's interests or fails to fulfil his role, the doctor is obliged to notify the court which may dismiss the agent and appoint a medical guardian in his place. The health care agent makes decisions to the extent that the patient would be entitled. Thus, just as in the case of a will autonomously expressed by the patient, the medical staff is not obligated to take actions requested by the agent that are contrary to medical indications. On the other hand, the medical staff is obliged to respect the agent's objection to the proposed medical action (Szeroczyńska et al. 2016a; 2016b). The appointed health care agent cannot make decisions within the scope that has been regulated by the patient in the form of a drafted living will statement. The patient's autonomy expressed directly *pro futuro* is placed higher than the decisions made by the health care agent. However, it should be mentioned that the issue of the functioning of living will statements in the Polish healthcare system and legal standards has not been clearly regulated either (Szeroczyńska 2004; Szeroczyńska et al. 2016a).

Attempts to normalize the legal basis for the functioning of health care agent were also made in the draft amendment to the Act on Patients'

Rights and the Ombudsman of Patients' Rights (Projekt nowelizacji Ustawy o Prawach Pacjenta i Rzeczniku Praw Pacjenta 2018). According to the provisions of this draft, any person who is at least 18 years old and not under guardianship may appoint another adult and not under guardianship as his health care agent. The appointment of a health care agent requires the written consent of the person appointed. It is possible to appoint only one agent, but it is possible to appoint someone else to be the agent in case the originally appointed agent is unable to take up his role for any reason (however, once these reasons cease and the agent takes up his role, the power of attorney for the alternative agent expires). If both the agent and any other person appointed to act in place of the agent are unable to perform their role, the patient will be deemed not to have a health care agent. The power of attorney should be in writing (certified by a notary public or by the mayor). The health care agent has the right to access information about the patient that is subject to medical confidentiality. The health care agent is obliged to act in the best interests of the patient and to keep confidential all information concerning the principal's health that is disclosed to him in relation to the power of attorney (Projekt nowelizacji Ustawy o Prawach Pacjenta i Rzeczniku Praw Pacjenta 2018).

The introduction of legal solutions normalizing the issues of health care agents was also requested by the Ombudsman. In letters to the Minister of Health, he pointed out that the existing regulations inadequately protect the autonomy of patients who are incapable of providing informed consent and at the same time do not have a legal representative. For this reason it is considered important to take legislative action to create solutions favorable to the protection of the will for this group of patients. An important step towards broadening the protection of patient rights and autonomy of incompetent patients and those without a statutory representative should be the legal regulation of *pro futuro* statements (Rzecznik Praw Obywatelskich 2018; 2020; 2021). Unfortunately, the declaration of the Ministry of Health to undertake work on the regulation of this issue has not yet resulted in the presentation of proposals for specific legal solutions (Rzecznik Praw Obywatelskich 2021).

Conclusions

Advance care planning allows patients to make decisions regarding their future care and treatment. As a part of *pro futuro* care planning, it is possible to appoint a health care agents to make decisions on behalf of the incompetent patients based on their preferences, beliefs and values.

Functioning of the institution of health care agent in Poland is primarily determined by the existing legal status—despite attempts made by medical and legal circles, there are still no regulations governing the functioning of health care agents as well as other forms of advance care planning. It is necessary to introduce into the current legal system clear regulations that would standardize the functioning of both health care agents and other forms of *pro futuro* declarations. Adoption of such solutions would strengthen the protection of patients' rights to self-determination, in areas related to medical care provided to them, in cases of loss of the actual ability to provide consent. It also seems reasonable to conduct a social information campaign on issues related to advance care planning. The information should be directed to patients, potential patients and their relatives, as well as to medical personnel.

References

Aasmul I., Husebo B., Flo E. 2018. Description of an advance care planning intervention in nursing homes: outcomes of the process evaluation. *BMC Geriatrics* 18(1): 26.

Bomba P. 2017. Supporting the patient voice: Building the foundation of shared decision-making. *Generations* 41(1): 21–30.

Boerner K., Carr D., Moorman S. 2013. Family relationships and advance care planning: Do supportive and critical relations encourage or hinder planning? *The Journal of Gerontology Series B: Psychological Sciences and Social Sciences* 68(2): 246–256.

Brown B. 2003. The history of advance directives. A literature review. *Journal of Gerontological Nursing* 29(9): 4–14.

Buckey J., Molina O. 2012. Honoring patient care preferences: surrogates speak. *Omega (Westport)* 65(4): 257–280.

Carr D., Luth E. 2017. Advance care planning: Contemporary issues and future directions. *Innovation in Aging* 28(1): igx012.

Carr D., Luth E. 2019. Well-being at the end of life. *Annual Review of Sociology* 45: 515–534.

Cheng S., Lin C., Chan H., Martina D., Mori M., Kim H., Ng R. 2020. Advance care planning in Asian culture. *Japanese Journal of Clinical Oncology* 50(9): 976–989.

Council of Europe. 2009. *Principles concerning continuing powers of attorney and advance directives for incapacity.* Recommendation CM/Rec (2009) 11 adopted by the Committee of Ministers of the Council of Europe on 09 December 2009 and explanatory memorandum. Council of Europe Publishing, Strasbourg 2011. Available at: https://rm.coe.int/168070965f. Accessed: 20.12.2017.

Detering K., Hancock A., Reade M., Silvester W. 2010. The impact of advance care planning on end-of-life care in elderly patients: Randomised controlled trial. *BMJ (Clinical research ed.)* 340: c1345.

Dunlay S., Strand J. 2016. How to discuss goals of care with patients. *Trends in Cardiovascular Medicine* 26(1): 36–43.

Escher M., Perneger T., Rudaz S., Dayer P., Perrier A. 2014. Impact of advance directives and a health care proxy on doctors' decisions: A randomized trial. *Journal of Pain and Symptom Management* 47(1): 1–11.

Fritsch J., Petronio S., Helft P., Torke A. 2013. Making decisions for hospitalized older adults: Ethical factors considered by family surrogates. *Journal of Clinical Ethics* 24(2): 125–134.

Grądalski T., Kochan K. 2017. Incompetent terminal patients' key carers expectations. *Medycyna Paliatywna* [*Palliative Medicine*] 9(1): 21–29.

Grzejszczak R., Szeroczyńska M. 2012. Praktyka wyrażania zgody zastępczej za pacjentów faktycznie niekompetentnych: Raport z badań. *Człowiek – Niepełnosprawność – Społeczeństwo* 4: 87–108.

Hamilton I. 2017. Advance care planning in general practice: Promoting patient autonomy and shared decision making. *The British Journal of General Practice: the Journal of the Royal College of General Practitioners* 67(656): 104–105.

Korfage I., Carreras G., Arnfeldt Christensen C., Billekens P., Bramley L. et al. 2020. Advance care planning in patients with advanced cancer: A 6-country, cluster-randomised clinical trial. *PLoS Medicine* 17(11): e1003422.

Kim H., Deatrick J., Ulrich C. 2017. Ethical frameworks for surrogates' end-of-life planning experiences. *Nursing Ethics* 24(1): 46–69.

Luck T., Rodriguez F., Wiese B., van der Leeden C., Heser K., Bickel H. et al. 2017. Advance directives and power of attorney for health care in the oldest-old—results of the AgeQualiDe study. *BMC Geriatrics* 17(1): 85.

Luck H., Dukes J., Church S., Abbott J., Youngwerth J. 2018. Teaching medical students about "The Conversation": An interactive value-based advance care planning session. *American Journal of hospice & Palliative Care* 35(2): 324–329.

McMahan R., Knight S., Fried T., Sudore R. 2013. Advance care planning beyond advance directives: Perspectives from patients and surrogates. *Journal of Pain and Symptom Management* 46(3): 355–365.

Michael N., O'Callaghan C., Sayers E. 2017. Managing 'shades of grey': A focus group study exploring community-dwellers' views on advance care planning in older people. *BMC Palliative Care,* 16(1): 2.

Montanari Vergallo G. 2020. Advance healthcare directives: Binding or informational value? *Cambridge Quarterly of Healthcare Ethics: CQ: The International Journal of Healthcare Ethics Committees* 29(1): 98–109.

Mullick A., Martin J., Sallnow L. 2013. An introduction to advance care planning in practice. *BMJ (Clinical research ed.)* 347: f6064.

Naczelna Rada Lekarska. 2016. *Stanowisko nr 19/16/VII Naczelnej Rady Lekarskiej w sprawie stworzenia w polskim prawie instytucji pełnomocnika medycznego.* Available at: https://sip.lex.pl/akty-prawne/akty-korporacyjne/stworzenie-w-polskim-prawie-instytucji-pelnomocnika-medycznego-286958915. Accessed: 15.02.2021.

Pawłowski L., Modlińska A., Lichodziejewska-Niemierko M. 2019. Selected aspects of advance careplanning according to Polish legal regulations—physician's requirements. *Palliative Medicine in Practice* 13(4): 197–203.

Prince-Paul M., DiFranco E. 2017. Upstreaming and normalizing advance care planning conversations—a public health approach. *Behavioral Sciences (Basel)* 7(2): E18.

Projekt nowelizacji Ustawy o Prawach Pacjenta i Rzeczniku Praw Pacjenta oraz niektórych innych ustaw. 2013. Available at: https://hospicjum.waw.pl/pliki/Artykul/1364_projekt-ustawy-o-zmianie-ustawy-o-prawach-pacjenta-i-rzecznikupraw-pacjenta.pdf. Accessed: 15.02.2021.

Projekt nowelizacji Ustawy o Prawach Pacjenta i Rzeczniku Praw Pacjenta. 2018. Available at: https://archiwum.rpp.gov.pl/gfx/bpp/userfiles/_public/akty_prawne/nowelizacja_ustawy2018.pdf. Accessed: 10.02.2021.

Potter J., Lee S. 2020. When advance directives collide. *Journal of General Internal Medicine* 35(7): 2191–2192.

Rzecznik Praw Obywatelskich. 2018. Pismo do Ministra Zdrowia z dnia 5.03.2018. Available at: https://www.rpo.gov.pl/sites/default/files/RPO%20do%20MZ%20w%20sprawie%20pe%C5%82nomocnictwa%20medycznego.pdf. Accessed: 15.02.2021.

Rzecznik Praw Obywatelskich. 2020. *Dylematy prawa i bioetyki – pora na działanie. Stanowiska i postulaty Rzecznika Praw Obywatelskich dotyczące problemów bioetycznych w czasie VII kadencji (2015–2020)*, 7–12. Warszawa: Wydawnictwo Rzecznika Praw Obywatelskich. Available at: https://www.rpo.gov.pl/sites/default/files/DYLEMATY_PRAWA_i_BIOETYKI.pdf. Accessed: 15.02.2011.

Rzecznik Praw Obywatelskich. 2021. Pismo do Ministra zdrowia z dnia 05.02.2021. Available at: https://www.rpo.gov.pl/sites/default/files/Do_MZ_oswiadczenia_pro_futuro_5.02.2021.pdf. Accessed: 10.02.2021.

Rietjens J., Sudore R., Connolly M., van Delden J., Drickamer M., Droger M. et al. 2017. Definition and recommendations for advance care planning: an international consensus supported by the European Association for Palliative Care. *The Lancet Oncology* 18(9): e543–e551.

Rosoff P. 2017. Licensing surrogate decision-makers. *HEC Forum: An Interdisciplinary Journal on Hospitals' Ethical and Legal Issues* 29(2): 145–169.

Sinclair C., Auret K., Evans S., Williamson F., Dormer S., Wilkinson A. et al. 2017. Advance care planning uptake among patients with severe lung disease: A randomised patient preference trial of a nurse-led, facilitated advance care planning intervention. *BMJ Open* 7(2): e013415.

Schellinger S., Anderson E., Frazer M., Cain C. 2018. Patient self-defined goals: Essentials of person-centered care for serious illness. *The American Journal of Hospice and Palliative Care* 35(1): 159–165.

Sudore R., Fried T. 2010. Redefining the "planning" in advance care planning: Preparing for end-of-life decision making. *Annals of Internal Medicine* 153(4): 256–261.

Sudore R., Lum H., You J., Hanson L., Meier D., Pantilat S. et al. 2017a. Defining advance care planning for adults: A consensus definition from a multidisciplinary delphi panel. *Journal of Pain and Symptom Management* 53(5): 821–832.

Sudore R., Heyland D., Barnes D., Howard M., Fassbender K., Robinson C. et al. 2017b. Measuring advance care planning: Optimizing the advance care planning engagement survey. *Journal of Pain and Symptom Management* 53(4): 669–681.e8.

Sulmasy D., Hughes M., Yenokyan G., Kub J., Terry P., Astrow A., Johnson J.A., Ho G., Nolan M.T. 2017. The trial of ascertaining individual preferences for loved ones' role in end-of-life decisions (TAILORED) study: A randomized controlled trial to improve surrogate decision making. *Journal of Pain Symptom Management* 54(4): 455–465.

Sussman T., Kaasalainen S., Bui M., Akhtar-Danesh N., Mintzberg S., Strachan P. 2017. "Now I don't have to guess:" using pamphlets to encourage residents and families/friends to engage in advance care planning in long-term care. *Gerontology and Geriatric Medicine* 3: 2333721417747323.

Szeroczyńska M. 2004. *Eutanazja i wspomagane samobójstwo na świecie*. Kraków: Universitas.

Szeroczyńska M. 2013. Dopuszczalność uprzednich oświadczeń pacjenta i pełnomocnictwa medycznego *de lege lata* i *de lege ferenda*. Available at: https://hospicjum.waw.pl/pliki/Artykul/1105_dopuszczalnosc-uprzednich-oswiadczen-pacjenta-i-pelnomocnictwa-medycznego-de-lege-lata-i-de-lege-ferenda.pdf. Accessed: 12.02.2021.

Szeroczyńska M., Czarkowski M., Krajnik M., Krajewski R., Pawłowski L., Adamczyk A. et al. 2016a. Instytucja pełnomocnika medycznego w Polsce – stanowisko Polskiej Grupy Roboczej ds. Problemów Etycznych Końca Życia. *Medycyna Praktyczna* 5: 102–112.

Szeroczyńska M., Czarkowski M., Krajnik M., Krajewski R., Pawłowski L., Adamczyk A. et al. 2016b. Institution of health care agent in Polish legislation: Position of the Polish Working Group on End-of-Life ethics. *Polskie Archiwum Medycyny Wewnętrznej* 126(5): 313–320.

Torke A., Sachs G., Helft P., Montz K., Hui S., Slaven J., Callahan Ch.M. 2014. Scope and outcomes of surrogate decision making among hospitalized older adults. *JAMA Intern Medicine* 174(3): 370–377.

Quenot J.P., Ecarnot F., Meunier-Beillard N., Dargent A., Large A., Andreu P., Rigaud J.Ph. 2017. What are the ethical questions raised by the integration of intensive care into advance care planning? *Annals of Translational Medicine 5(Suppl 4)*: S46.

Ustawa o zawodach lekarza i lekarza dentysty. Dz.U. 1997 Nr 28, poz. 152 z późniejszymi zmianami. Available at: http://isap.sejm.gov.pl/isap.nsf/download.xsp/WDU19970280152/U/D19970152Lj.pdf. Accessed: 10.02.2020.

Ustawa o prawach pacjenta i Rzeczniku praw pacjenta. Dz.U. 2009 Nr 52 poz. 417 z późniejszymi zmianami. Available at: http://isap.sejm.gov.pl/isap.nsf/download.xsp/WDU20090520417/U/D20090417Lj.pdf. Accessed: 10.02.2021.

Vig E., Taylor J., Starks H., Hopley E., Fryer-Edwards K. 2006. Beyond substituted judgment: How surrogates navigate end-of-life decision-making. *Journal of the American Geriatrics Society*, 54(11): 1688–1693.

Vig E., Taylor J., O'Hare A. 2017. Considering a family systems approach to surrogate decision-making. *Families, Systems & Health: The Journal of Collaborative Family Healthcare* 35(1): 85–87.

Waszkiewicz K. 2017. Pełnomocnictwo medyczne w świetle obowiązujących przepisów ustawowych. *Rynek - Społeczeństwo - Kultura* 26: 133–136.

Wendler D. 2017. The theory and practice of surrogate decision-making. *The Hastings Center Report* 47(1): 29–31.

Ethical Aspects of Patient Autonomy

Valery Sokolchik

Respecting the Autonomy of the Dying Patient

Abstract

The article focuses on the autonomy of the dying patient as expressed in the right to know the truth about their illness and prognosis, the right to receive support, understanding and respect, as well as the right to make own decisions about their life and death. In brief, the main theme is respect for the dying patient's autonomy.

It can be safely said that most physicians are not taught how to communicate the truth to dying patients. Some doctors opt for a paradigm in which the opinion, feelings, desires of dying people are not taken into account in the struggle for life. This paternalist point of view sometimes involves manipulating a dying person's hope through meaningless acts undertaken against death. Informed consent (and other legal instruments) can be a legitimate way of explaining the situation to a dying patient if we are willing to discuss the alternatives to treatment.

Special training courses for medical staff should highlight ideas and techniques that will enable them to respect the wishes and values of a dying man, learning how to "listen correctly" and manifest empathy.

Keywords: autonomy, respect, dying patient, healthcare workers, informed consent, ethical skills, empathy, values, "to say the truth," DNR, palliative care

Introduction

Approximately 56 million people die around the world each year. Of this total more than 50% perish from cardiovascular disease, cancer, infections, etc. That is why discussions about death as an ethical phenomenon and disputes over the feelings, emotions and thoughts of the dying are very significant and remarkable for many people in our society, including medical professionals, patients facing death, their relatives and other interested parties.

Every country has a great number of dying people who need medical, psychological, and legal help. And most of this help and support comes from health care providers. When considering the dying patient's autonomy medical professionals, and all members of the caring profession are not only required to make every effort to reduce the patient's pain, but also to provide information, communicate with the patient, find legal solutions to ambiguous problems, and act as therapists and psychologists (Yahanda 2020).

Our ethical discussions with both medical professionals at the Belarusian Medical Academy of Postgraduate Education (BelMAPE) and with patients revealed clear psychological, legal and communication gaps in the relationship between health care providers and dying patients.

This article highlights importance of the dying patient's autonomy as the foundation of the respect and understanding that every human being deserves.

Patient autonomy in end-of-life care

The autonomy of the dying patient will be considered to encompass the following: the right to know the truth about illness, the right to be informed of their prognosis and life expectancy, the right to receive support, understanding and respect, and also the right to make decisions about their own life and death.

Respecting and enforcing the dying patient's autonomy is closely connected with ensuring the patient is aware of truth regarding their diagnosis and life expectancy. Most physicians are not taught how to communicate the truth (bad news) to dying patients (Balaban 2000; Bernacki and Block 2014). Sometimes a conversation with a dying patient becomes a serious problem and this dialogue is not based on the important principle of medical ethics, i.e, the duty to "to tell the truth." We understand that truth can be very powerful weapon in the fight for life, in which the doctor and the dying patient are both participants. From my point of view, telling the truth in a transparent way that ensures protection and respect, is absolutely essential for encouraging the autonomous patient to take responsibility for their life and wellbeing. When informing the patient of their diagnosis, risks and prognosis the physician requires special psychological and ethical skills (Balaban 2000; Balea et al. 2000). In the BelMAPE, we organized training courses dealing with different social, ethical and psychological aspects of health care, including communication skills (including "Bioethical Aspects of Communication in the Healthcare System," "The Ethical and Psychological Competences of the Doctor," "The Culture of Social Communication," "Ethical and legal questions connected with the practical activity of Ethical Committees"). The topics discussed in these training courses are broader in scope and more voluminous than simply teaching the ability to talk with patients. This experience can be considered in the context of the fact that training courses are the basic foundation of a physician's professional social skills, including communicating the truth to the dying patient.

Different countries have different paradigms for teaching healthcare providers the skills needed to "tell the truth," make difficult ethical decisions, etc. For example, some medical professionals prefer training, while others opt for round-table discussions with their colleagues on issues, and yet others favour special postgraduate courses. These are all very productive methods, and every healthcare system has developed a viable and rewarding learning option for its needs and every healthcare provider should take advantage of the opportunity and need to promote, learn and develop psychological and ethical skills.

In light of the ethical principles of patient autonomy and the need to communicate the truth, the paternalistic approach to the patient should be called into question. The latter approach has negative consequences for the dying patient (Beauchamp and Childress 2012; Sokolchik 2017). The most common allegory to such a situation would be the interaction between a wise teacher and a young pupil where the teacher chooses the correct path of life for his pupil even if the latter is an autonomous adult person who prefers to make choices on his own account. There is a discrepancy between the views and values of the doctor and the patient, and, as a result, there is a discrepancy between their different positions when it comes decisions regarding life and health.

For example, some doctors adopt a paradigm in which the fight to preserve life does not take into account the opinions, feelings, desires and financial capabilities of people facing death. The paternalist perspective sometimes involves manipulating the dying person's hopes through meaningless actions against illness and death. The serious problems entailed by such paternalist pressure exerted on the patient have been described by Kate McLean in her emotional article "Doctors need to talk about death instead of trying to keep patients alive at any cost" (McLean 2020). According to Kate McLean, "patients who are provided with complete information about their prognosis and treatment options elect to have less intervention than those placed on the 'default treatment path.'" A recent physician poll showed that, while doctors believe it's their responsibility to provide this information through end-of-life conversations, only approximately 30% have had some formal training in doing so. Doctors are therefore reluctant to have these conversations, even when their patients are severely ill" (McLean 2020).

There are genuine negative consequences (both ethical and legal) when a doctor, in a desire to be a "good person" discusses the dying patient's poor prognosis with their relatives without the consent of the patient and in spite of their duty to maintain medical confidentiality. Though legally prohibited in most countries of the world, such practices are common. With the well-being of the patient in mind doctors sometimes violate the patient's legal and ethical ownership of personal data, including by disclosing to others their diagnosis and the prospects of possible treatment. Discussing the patient's condition without his (her) consent should be classified as a harmful breach of medical ethics, law and medical professional practice; perhaps this undermines respect for the patient, transparency of the doctor-patient relationship, as well as trust in the medical profession in general. In any case, healthcare providers cannot rely on their psychological sense of the situation only. They cannot know the internal feelings of all the participants involved. That is why doctors have to avoid breaking ethical (legal) rules. The right approach for medical professionals in such cases is to engage in personal communication with the patient or (if the patient does not wish to talk to the doctor about his illness, prognosis, etc.) obtain the patient's consent to talk to his (her) relatives (Council of Europe Guide 2014).

In actual practice informed consent can be a legitimate way to explain the circumstances of the disease and treatment for the dying patient if we are willing to debate the treatment alternatives. Ensuring that decision-making is based on legal foundations and expressed in a legal document would be a useful means of resolving the situation and guaranteeing a productive conversation between the doctor and the patient (Tretyakov 2019; Walker 2008).

One important issue regarding the autonomy of a dying patient is the legal mechanisms that ensure that the legal order "do not resuscitate" (DNR) is respected. Considering the ethical ambiguity of this order in real situations the preferable approach is to follow Article 9 of the Oviedo Convention (regarding previously expressed wishes): "The previously expressed wishes relating to a medical intervention by a patient who is not at the time of the intervention in a state to express his or her wishes shall be taken into account" (Council of Europe Convention 1997).

In Belarus we do not have the legal means to enforce the patient's refusal to be resuscitated. According to established practice, dying patients have the right to leave a written DNR declaration, but in cases involving acute medical care such a note or declaration will not be deemed legitimate when set alongside the Criminal Code, which requires medical professionals to save lives and provide urgent medical assistance. That is why medical staff working in an Intensive Care Unit (ICU) know very well that the patient's will is only a "right on paper" and this right does not correlate with actual DNR. "Saving lives" may be the declared slogan of the medical profession, but such "lives" are only an abstract term. These lives are cut off from their carriers, from the will of autonomous patients.

The next step to enforcing the dying patient's autonomy is to foster a close connection between the doctor, the patient and palliative care, which sometimes appears to be genuine way to help and improve the conditions of people facing the prospect of death.

Every person needs to be aware that palliative care is not a precursor of death. It can be defined as a way of helping achieve normal quality of life without pain and fear. Every dying patient has the right to be relieved of the pain that is associated with disease, including by having access to special pain relief medications in outpatient-care at home.

By means of palliative care, the dying patient has the chance to place the focus of care on quality of life, obtain help in coping with suffering and (perhaps above all else) not be alone at the time of death.

Three steps to informed consent

After taking into account the best practices around the world that respect the will of the patient., we formulated three steps (three conclusions) for ensuring legitimate informed consent. The first step involves determining who will be informed about the patient's illness and who will sign the informed consent (i.e., who will be deemed the autonomous persons).[1] If the consent form features the signature of the dying patient's legal representative or guardian rather than that of the dying patient him or herself, our focus should be on defending the non-autonomous person's interests and determining his (her) own will. The second step consists in scrutinizing the full content and legal status of the informed consent document (I mean here, the document should be jointly considered by both the doctor and the patient). And the third step is to ensure that there is sufficient time to read the document, and that it can be read in comfortable conditions and without any pressure. Familiarizing oneself with informed consent takes time—the patient needs to think it over, obtain clarification and advice, before making a decision. An important factor when signing a consent form is to ensure a calm and, if possible, comfortable environment, as well as maintain confidentiality, and prevent any pressure and coercion. Coercion and pressure are not necessarily expressed in words. The patient is often placed in a situation (due to lack of time or being presented with the "consequences" of their immediate failure to sign

[1] In our case this person is the dying patient or his (her) legal representative.

the papers) where sometimes he or she signs an informed consent without understanding it.

Respecting the wishes of the patient for a comfortable environment and providing them with enough time to read and sign an informed consent form is very difficult to guarantee in some modern healthcare establishments. Objectively speaking, here is not always a room available where the doctor can calmly discuss informed consent with the patient. Subjective reasons usually include a lack of time, an unwillingness (inability) to answer "endless questions," and, in general, the cold, formal approach of the doctor to the signing process.

Despite all the difficulties of both an objective and subjective nature, each medical professional must remember that once they are in the patient's place, they will look at the problem completely differently, wishing to get as much information as possible and discuss it with the doctor (or other persons). Perhaps he or she (the medical professional) will react negatively to any manifestation of pressure (Tran and Angelos 2020).

As in all countries, palliative care in Belarus is one of the most specific and helpful sources of support available to the dying patient. It is an area that requires improving in the current healthcare system. Palliative care was first introduced in Belarus in 1994 with the opening of its first children's hospice. A year later a "hospice" for adult patients was built in Minsk, and a definition of "palliative care" was incorporated into the country's Healthcare Law. Currently, the country has 463 palliative beds in in-patient hospitals, 18 palliative beds in out-patient clinics and hospitals, 15 palliative care clinics, 10 units providing home palliative care, etc. These facilities are probably insufficient for the needs of our country, because more than 75,000 patients in Belarus need palliative care nowadays.

When discussing the palliative care system in a modern society, we should also be aware of the great potential and training of palliative care professionals. Given the growing numbers of patients, palliative care is needed all over the world. The experiences of current palliative care professionals should be taken into account when considering howe to provide palliative care in different places (for example, in rural areas, where there are few hospices) and special training courses and workshops in palliative care are required for for family doctors, nurses, volunteers, etc.

Palliative care normally comes down to offering a "helping hand" to the dying patient, and one of the main tasks of palliative care is to ensure patients quality of life and offer them adequate and possible resources appropriate to the current situation, including information. It is also a way of respecting the autonomy of the dying patient. Every country, every official palliative care system usually tries to create different resources (for example, sites, YouTube channels) for people in need of care and guardianship. In accordance with good practice, these information platforms post useful advice for dying people in the form of psychological support, information on different volunteer projects, communication supportive opportunities, schedules for palliative staff, etc. In Belarus, we also have special red cross units and hospices, where patients and their relatives can find various forms of care (https://redcross.by/, http://www.mhospice.of.by/, https://hospice.by/ru/index.php/). However, improving the quality and quantity of information resources is required.

Conclusions

In this paper we considered the most important ethical, legal, psychological and communication issues connected with the autonomy of the dying patient, and our final conclusions will be presented in the form of a short list of both general and specific ethical principles and rules of interpersonal communication for medical staff, including doctors.

The general list of rules for dealing with dying patients is based on the following issues:

1. Respect the patient's needs and views (do not try and stress your own values, experiences and perception of the problem):
   a) show respect for the dignity, autonomy and different values of the patient as well as support their desire for independence;
   b) people may have different religions, try to respect their need for prayer;
   c) be aware of the fact that elderly people may take things at a slower pace (Solojenkin 1997);
   d) communicate with the patient in a respectful manner (i.e., how do they like to be addressed? What barriers are there to communication?);
   e) understand that each individual has different needs: patience, tolerance, kindness, understanding, empathy, encouragement, support, etc. (Stewart et al. 2000);
   f) don't use time pressure or workload as a reason for not showing respect.
2. Respect the patient's decision, if they deliberately/consciously refuse help: every person, every human being prefers to decide for themself about their own life and wishes based on their own values and dreams and we cannot overlook their preferences and hopes (Williams et al. 2014).
3. Tell patients the truth.

4. Ensure that the dying patient's consent has been obtained before talking to their relatives about their diagnosis, treatment, prognosis, etc.
5. Encourage the patient to communicate with their loved ones (Walker 2008). This conversation seems to be the best medicine for a dying person and the most successful therapy available. Love creates new hope and talking with one's loved ones slows down the illness.
6. Show empathy and be a "good listener." Empathy is often described as "putting yourself in someone else's shoes," and it's about listening to what's going on in our patients' minds. Another side of psychological compassion is sympathy. Sympathy can be more about managing your own feelings than understanding the situation and feelings of the dying patient. To show empathy, the first thing the carer should do is try to understand what someone is going through from their point of view (Batt-Rawden et al. 2013; Hojat et al. 2002). Researchers have observed "a significant postintervention increase in empathy, which suggests that empathy is a skill that can be modified by educational strategies" (Yahanda 2020). The first step to increasing empathy is being a good listener. If you listen carefully to what people say you can clarify your understanding by repeating back, summarising or reflecting on what you feel they are trying to communicate (Atwater 1992; Harvard Manage Mentor-coaching tools 2004). This skill includes verbal and non-verbal elements, and thus in addition to being a good active listener different factors should also be considered, such as appropriate body gestures and posture demonstrating engagement, as well as facial expressions, eye contact, showing interest in the speaker's words, minimum verbal encouragement, attentive silence, reflecting back feelings and content, and summarizing intellectually the speaker's words and their purpose (Robertson 2005; Stewart et al. 2000; Walker 2008). Active listening does not come naturally to most of us, and, like other communication skills, it must be learned and developed. Hence, as Jahromi argues, strategies need to be developed to ensure greater awareness among hospital managers of the importance of active listening skills (Jahromi et al. 2016).
7. Ensuring that the patient's right to be informed is respected. Try to make sure you have all the possible information that the patient may need (Roter et al. 1997). Firstly, this should include details about medical (or palliative care) resources (where and when can the patient get help in terms of health care, medicine, pain relief, etc.). Secondly, it should include information about where and when the patient can learn more about alternative treatment, statistics regarding their illness and the prognosis for their illness, etc.). Thirdly, there should be information regarding possible psychological and social support (when

and where can the patient get help from their local community, from various social organizations and free volunteers).

The specific rules for medical professionals may consist of the following tips:

a) do not make assumptions about how people are feeling or how they like to be treated;
b) take a realistic view of the circumstances;
c) do not say that everything will be fine (okay);
d) do not express a peremptory verdict (assertion);
e) set boundaries and time limits (medical professionals must observe this final rule so as to make sure they can reserve time for patients and prevent burnout) (Jahromi et al. 2016; Sokolchik 2017; Solojenkin 1997).

Understanding the patient's autonomy as a human right (and not only as the autonomy of a dying patient), learning the relevant skills, and showing patients respect constitute major challenges in modern medicine not only for health care providers, but also for (bio)ethical committees (commissions) in health establishments. The members of these (bio)ethical institutes should pay close attention to the importance of teaching staff about ethical issues and developing as well as implementing a collective decision-making algorithm for difficult situations. In this way the knowledge learned from the article "How should shared decision making be taught" (Tran and Angelos 2020) can be applied in real practice.

It ought to be emphasized that the capacity to respect the dying patient's autonomy is closely bound up with the ability to effectively manage such situations through the possession of ethical, legal, and psychological skills that a health care professional should possess. These skills and ethical steps require the simultaneous mobilization of public health resources (research, practice, and policy making), mainly with the aim of encouraging a private response to such situations, as well as a need to develop specific capabilities shaping policy and decision-making in line with local and regional needs and practices within the wider context of international/global experience and best practices.

References

Atwater E. 1992. *I Hear You: A Listening Skills Handbook* (Rev. Sub edition). New York: Walker and Co.

Balaban R. 2000. A physician's guide to talking about end-of-life care. *Journal of General Internal Medcine* 15(3): 195–200. Available at: https://www.ncbi.nlm.nih.gov/pmc/articles/PMC1495357. Accessed: 15.05.2020.

Balea W., Buckman R., Lenzi R. 2000. SPIKES—A six step protocol for dealing bad news: Application to the patient with cancer. *The Oncologist* 5: 43302–43311.

Batt-Rawden S.A., Chisolm M.S., Anton B., Flickinger T.E. 2013. Teaching empathy to medical students: an updated, systematic review. *Academic Medicine* 88(8): 1171–1177.

Beauchamp T.L., Childress J.F. 2012. *Principles of Biomedical Ethics* (7th ed.). Oxford: Oxford University Press.

Bernacki R., Block S. 2014. Communication about serious illness care goals: A review and synthesis of best practices. *JAMA Internal Medicine* 174(12): 1994–2003.

Council of Europe Convention for the protection of Human Rights and Dignity of the Human Being with regard to the Application of Biology and Medicine: Convention on Human Rights and Biomedicine (ETS No 164). 1997. Available at: https://www.coe.int/en/web/conventions/full-list/-/conventions/rms/090000168007cf98. Accessed: 15.07.2020.

Council of Europe Guide on the decision-making process regarding medical treatment in end-of-life situations. 2014. Available at: https://rm.coe.int/CoERMPublicCommonSearchServices/DisplayDCTMContent?documentId=090000168039e8c5. Accessed: 15.07.2020.

Harvard Manage Mentor-coaching tools. Active Listening Self-Assessment. 2004. Available at: http://www.mheducation.ca/college/mcshane4/student/olc/4obm_sa_08.html. Accessed: 15.07.2017.

Hojat M., Gonnella J.S., Nasca T.J., Mangione S., Vergare M., Magee M. 2002. Physician empathy: Definition, components, measurement, and relationship to gender and specialty. *American Journal of Psychiatry* 159(9): 1563–1569.

Jahromi V.K., Tabatabaee S.S., Abdar Z.E., Rajabi M. 2016. Active listening: The key of successful communication in hospital managers. *Electronic Physician* 8(3): 2123–2128. Available at: http://dx.doi.org/10.19082/2123. Accessed: 12.05.2017.

McLean K. 2020. Doctors need to talk about death instead of trying to keep patients alive at any cost. *HuffPost Personal.* Available at: https://www.huffpost.com/entry/doctors-talking-to-patients-death_n_5e272d2dc5b63211761a5c30. Accessed: 24.01.2020.

Robertson K. 2005. Active listening: More than just paying attention. *Australian Family Physician* 34(12): 1053–1055.

Roter D.L., Stewart M., Putname S.M., Lipkin M.J., Stiles W., Inui T.S. 1997. Communication patterns of primary care physicians. *JAMA* 277: 350–356.

Sokolchik V.N. 2017. Ethical aspect of communicative interaction between physician and patient. *Healthcare* 9: 34–39 (in Russian).

Solojenkin,V.V. 1997. Psychological foundations of medical practice. Available at: https://drive.google.com/file/d/1lVt_Y1TdYzB1ueqfSRZV7EcAMG45Gjjk/view (in Russian) Accessed: 15.07.2020.

Stewart M., Brown J.B., Donner A., McWhinney I.R., Oates J., Weston W.W., Jordan J. 2000. The impact of patient-centered care on outcomes. *Journal of Family Practice* 49(9): 796–804.

Tran D.K., Angelos P. 2020. How should shared decision making be taught? *AMA Journal of Ethics* 22(95): E388–394.

Tretyakov, D. 2019. The principle of informed consent in the practice of the European Court of Human Rights. *Case-law of the European Court of Himan Rights (Human Rights and Biomedicine).* Special Issue 14–16. (in Russian)

Walker R.L. 2008. The psychosocial and mental health of people who are affected by conflict, catastrophes, terrorism, adversity and displacement. In *Conflict and Catastrophe Medicine*, eds. J.M. Ryan, A.P.C.C. Hopperus Buma, C.W. Beadling, A. Mozumder, D.M. Nott, N.M. Rich, W. Henny, D. MacGarty, 805–849. London: Springer.

Williams R., Kemp V.J., Alexander D.A. 2014. The psychosocial and mental health of people. *Journal of Medicine and Philosophy* 33(6): 594–608.

Yahanda A.T. 2020. The importance of sharing health decisions. *AMA Journal of Ethics* 22(5): E349–351.

Marta Szabat

Parental Autonomy in the Light of Hope in Pediatric Palliative Care

Abstract

The article examines the language used by Health Care Professionals' (HCPs) during interpersonal communication with parents, in particular when discussing prenatal diagnoses and possible pediatric palliative care during pregnancy and later parental care for children with various genetic conditions such as Trisomy 13 (Patau syndrome) or Trisomy 18 (Edwards syndrome) and other life-threatening illnesses. As has become clear from relevant studies, some of the terms used by HCPs may be perceived by parents as offensive and unfortunate (e.g., phrases such as "incompatible with life," "lethal," etc.). Hence, in view of the vulnerable position of parents and the important role played by communication in the therapeutic process and its impact on parents' well-being and their capacity to become autonomous and responsible for their own decisions and choices, this paper presents a number of possible solutions to these issues. The author concludes that the most effective communication strategy in the case of prenatal diagnoses is one that is personally oriented towards each individual parent, and which ensures that the information is neutral and understandable and addressed in the parents' own language. Such a mode of interpersonal communication should leave room for hope, which itself serves a supportive function in that it allows parents to cope with highly sensitive decisions.

Keywords: pediatrics, autonomy, parents, palliative care, hope, clinical communication

Introduction

The purpose of this study is to discuss the metaphors used in interpersonal communication between Health Care Professionals (HCPs) and parents in the context of prenatal diagnoses that may entail possible pediatric palliative care (PPC) both during pregnancy and in the form of parental care for children with various genetic conditions, such as Trisomy 13 (Patau syndrome) or Trisomy 18 (Edwards syndrome) and other life-threatening illnesses.

This paper is divided into two parts. In the first, the author discusses the concept of autonomy and the strategy of maintaining parental hope. The second part focuses on the optimum language that should be used when informing parents of the abnormalities of their future child, which takes into account the need to maintain hope.

At the very outset, it is vital that we underline the difficulties involved in measuring pain in palliative treatment based on several scales and various psychological methods (Feudtner et al. 2010; Kim et al. 2014; Rumpold et al. 2017) and the ways in which these correlations lend an individual and personal character to both factors, especially in palliative care (PC) where pain needs to be understood holistically, including in its physical, psychical and spiritual aspects (Brown et al. 2016; Friedrichsdorf and Bruera 2018; Mok et al. 2010; Saunders et al. 1995; Saunders 2006). Additionally, it is also necessary to differentiate between generalized hope and particular hope. The first type refers to hope for the future, without any particular expectations—this is an optimistic perspective with a faith in future events. The second type concerns more personal needs and expectations (Daneault et al. 2010, p. 2310). The first kind of hope may also be associated with personal religious belief systems, which can help people to feel more secure by minimizing anxiety and helping them better cope with diagnoses and treatment (Hasson-Ohayon and Galinsky 2009, pp. 525–533).

At a linguistic level, the word *hope* has four different aspects in English. Firstly, hope is used as a noun: I can have *a hope of something* or have *hope for something.* I also can experience *hopefulness*—a state of being full of hope. This meaning is related to specific personal feelings regarding one's future. However, the present is also important in this context. Being full of hope influences the current situation and a person's present condition. In addition, *having (a) hope* is connected with either having control or being afraid of losing it. The meaning of *living with hope* expresses expectations and future preferences. For example, in an Australian study, twenty-eight patients with less than three months to live according to their medical prognosis were studied in terms of their use of the word *hope.* Some of the patients used hope as a noun and in this meaning: "hope was consistently presented as an objectively existing entity, centered on a hope of cure, and associated with a negative future that was beyond the patient's control" (Eliott et al. 2009, p. 612). Secondly, *hope* is also employed as a verb, giving it a dynamic meaning that directly expresses expectations for other persons and the situational environment. This verb transcends the present to the future. In the Australian study mentioned above, some patients used hope as a verb. According to the authors, this tendency: "was typically seen as subjectively determined by the patient, referencing what was personally meaningful, and associated with the depiction of a future with positive aspects" (Eliott et al. 2009, p. 612). The meanings of *hoping for something* also depends on personal preferences. Another Canadian study points to a number of possibilities: "hoping for comfort, peace, families; for cure; realistic and desirable possibilities" (Duggleby et al. 2012, p. 1217). The third meaning of hope is conveyed through the adjective *hopeful*, which has three different uses: *hopeful + noun*, to be *hopeful about something*, or to be *hopeful of doing something*. The fourth sense of hope is conveyed in the adverb *hopefully*, used to directly express a person's expectations regarding the future (Oxford English Dictionary 2021). The English etymology of hope reveals at least two features of hope. Firstly, hope as a noun is closely tied to the present directed to the future and expresses a patient's need to control the situation, which, in fact, is impossible due to unpredictable changes in their own individual situations. Secondly, when someone hopes *for* something, the element of failure is contained within the dialectic of possibility *versus* impossibility. The dynamic character of hoping reveals that anything can happen, including unexpected and unwanted events. The adjective *hopeful* and adverb *hopefully* also signal every possible present or future action.

All the above-mentioned aspects of hope should be related to a personal autonomy, especially when it comes to decisions regarding palliative care or making choices during the palliative treatment. That is why in the next part of this article the meaning of autonomy will be discussed together with its links to maintaining parental hope.

Parental autonomy and holding on to hope

The idea of autonomy can be understood as a value, a capacity, a virtue, an advantage and even a kind of human right (Dworkin 1988; Beauchamp and Childress 2001). The traditional understanding of autonomy is based on rational and critical reason as determining a person's actions (in particular, Kant's categorical imperative), the primacy of the individual (John Stuart Mill's concept of freedom) as well as Pellegrino's concept of autonomy as a moral right exercised by patients and physicians—both sides being obligated to respect this right (Pellegrino 1994, p. 68). According to Pellegrino, autonomy and beneficence complement one another. Only in such a situation can autonomy be good and useful. However, there may also arise conflicts of interest, in which the autonomy of one person excludes the possibility of another's autonomy: "[...] in theory and in practice, autonomy is a positive as well as a negative principle" (Pellegrino 1994, p. 48). Continuing this line of thinking, the authors of *Principles of Biomedical Ethics* claim that autonomy can be achieved only to a certain extent. An autonomous decision is characterized by sufficient recognition of certain situations as well as a knowledge of the process, procedure, circumstances, prognosis, and consequences of one's planned actions (Beauchamp and Childress 2001). An awareness of the disadvantages specific to a situation is sufficient to make a decision autonomous. Knowledge of a particular situation helps the agent to calculate the risk, potential advantages or disadvantages and to make his or her own decisions.

In contrast to this reason-based understanding of autonomy, James Griffin argues that we cannot be fully autonomous; rather "we could express our ideal, instead, as coming as close to total impartiality as we can" (Griffin 2015, p. 42). The philosopher also notes: "Normative agency consists not only in deciding for oneself what is worth doing, but also in doing it" (Griffin 2008, p. 150). The normative status of agency determines the values constituting an agent's identity. Being autonomous means that an agent is capable of being responsible but, at the same time, even without being responsible, he or she remains autonomous on a normative and moral level. Autonomy is a part of Griffin's concept of personhood elaborated in terms of autonomy, liberty and a "minimum provision," understood as "life itself [...], a certain level of health, certain physical and mental capacities, a certain amount of education" (Griffin 2008, p. 149). Thus, according to Griffin, autonomy appears as both a capacity and a virtue understood as a different value from liberty. In this sense, the constraints of illness, the necessity of treatment and the impoverishment of quality of life in an end-of-life (EOL) state are not obstacles to maintaining patient autonomy. Rather, these factors can be interpreted as reducing personal liberty. Obstacles preventing a person from using his or her autonomy include: "indoctrination, brain-washing, domination, manipulation, conformity, conventionality, false consciousness, certain forms of immaturity" (Griffin 2008, p.151).

In the case of agents lacking full competence, such as embryos, foetuses, or children incapable of taking responsibility for their actions, it is possible to consider their autonomy in the broader context of informed consent standards, the agent's legal representation or responsibility within the framework of autonomy based on relationships, in which the agent's decisions are made in conjunction with others, e.g., the agent's loved ones (Walker and Lovat 2015, p. 321). In the latter situation, autonomy is understood as an interpersonal factor where empathy, relationships and proper communication play a key role in making autonomous decisions. The issue of incompetent agents shows how important it is to help agents when making these types of decisions and choices. According to Walker and Lovat, who further developed the concept *relational autonomy* elaborated by Mackenzie and Stoljar (2000),

> the moral decisions to be made, as the end-of-life approaches, are set in the context of this particular individual patient, considering their lived socio-cultural experience and the relationships they have, as well as the underlying clinical problem and stage of its natural history [...]; the dialogue [...] is properly grounded in these nuanced understandings of personhood and of autonomy. This dialogue is characterized by being inclusive, non-coercive and reflective (Walker and Lovat 2015, p. 313).

The most important values for this type of dialogue are freedom and equality—each participant has the right to have his/her preferences respected: "to reach consensus about what is best for the community which is having the dialogue" (Walker and Lovat 2015, p. 313). In this perspective, dialogue should be understood as a form of discussion and consensus-building.

It is worth noting that certain studies indicate that some patients find conversations on vulnerable issues are easier with professionals than with family members (Clayton et al. 2008; Stans et al. 2018). As a consequence, one of the most important issues when it comes to vulnerable decisions is not only how EOL care should be carried out but also when, where and also *with whom*. In some cases, when making decisions we must be aware of the risk of that harming someone for the sake of higher needs (e.g. the need to maintain a patient's hope at the cost of carefully choosing the right moment when to inform the patient about potentially harmful circumstances). That is the reason why good standards of communication must be based on knowledge, which in turn constitutes the foundation of the agent's actions and anticipation of the consequences. Thus, each care process is dynamic in form and should be formalized as a procedure in which parents who make decisions on behalf of their children can change their mind on health care and treatment issues whenever they want or need to regarding their child's best interests. On this point, the EOL care from a parental perspective can be difficult for all sides—parents, their loved ones and HCPs. In certain situations, parents and their loved ones may feel obligated to consider EOL issues regardless of their feelings and circumstances (e.g. parents' decisions in light of a prenatal diagnosis or decisions to terminate causal treatment of their child in order to start PC). On the other hand, medical staff should communicate with parents in ways which requires effort, patience and time. In this context intentional and planned actions should not only take into account medical issues but also to communication skills. Consequently, a patient's right to information can be understood both as a form of autonomy and a right to dignity as well as, from the perspective of Griffin's minimum provision, the right to receive a satisfactory level of care. Moreover, a patient's rights regarding their own state of health can be considered on at least three levels: firstly, as a practical basis, in the sense of accepted social habits in certain institutions and shared cultural rules; secondly, in terms of a patient's right regarding their personal and individual situation; thirdly on the normative level, as a set of universal, minimum standards, and as high priority norms (Cruft et al. 2015; Nickel 2007).

The vulnerable position of parents compared to HCPs leaves the former gives rise to inequality in interpersonal communication. This is the reason why HCPs cannot play the role of service providers in the economic sense of treating patients as clients. Ethical codes require medical staff to adopt an appropriate approach to patients in terms of providing verbal and non-verbal information based on a sense of fairness. This includes ensuring equal treatment for individuals finding themselves in unfortunate circumstances. Thus, the expectation of proper communication that enables the patient to maintain hope in present and future medical care ensures that a patient has a fair chance of being treated with dignity and respect. Moreover, such communication needs to be understood in terms of reciprocity with regard to parental needs. Maintaining an attitude of helpfulness and "being there for parents" can provide moral foundations for using communication as an additional tool in any medical treatment. Following the Hippocratic principle of medicine "first, do no harm," it is worth nothing that suitable communication makes it possible to avoid unnecessary harm and should constitute a valid skill for HCPs even though when their role is only to inform parents about abnormalities in pregnancy or co-ordinating PC for their children.

Parental right to be properly informed

According to various studies, parents need to cope with the following communication issues between themselves and HCPs: inadequate communication by HCPs of difficult information, including through the use of terms and phrases to identify children with variations of genetic conditions that parents may find unacceptable, such as Trisomy 13 (Patau syndrome) or Trisomy 18 (Edwards syndrome) (Janvier et al. 2012, p. 293). In this regard, noticeable is the repetition of terms such as "incompatible with life," "would live a life of suffering," "would be a vegetable," "would live a meaningless life," "would ruin their parents' marriage," "would ruin their family," "a waste of money/time/energy," "lethal," "there is nothing we can do for him/her," "you can have another one," "this child will hurt you/your family/your children" (Janvier et al. 2012, pp. 295–296; Szabat 2020, pp. 4–5, 7, 9). Parents who chose clinical intervention for their child also felt judged by HCPs (Janvier et al. 2012, p. 295).

The use of the terms quoted above could be interpreted by parents as offensive for several reasons. Firstly, parents find themselves in an unequal and highly vulnerable position in relation to HCPs. Hence, their dignity and well-being with regard to their future responsibility for their child's care is placed under threat. In situations where parents must be informed about congenital malformations or other serious illnesses of the fetus, the burden of the situation shifts to the attitudes that HCPs' adopt towards parents. Secondly, as was mentioned in the previous section, the basic principle of medical care is "first, do no harm." Moreover, in the Corpus Hippocraticus as well as in contemporary medical codes of ethics include many passages and sentences that reflect a deeply humanistic approach to medical care rooted not only in knowledge and practical or even technical skills but also in a love of the art of medicine, of patients and of humanity as a whole (Askitopoulou and Vgontzas 2018). Thirdly, when it comes to the parents' of seriously or terminally ill children the extent of any eventual harm needs to be considered individually, taking into account the particular situation of each family, because objective harm would be impossible to calculate. Furthermore, as many studies show, improper verbal and non-verbal communication has a negative impact on parents in such vulnerable situations (Janvier et al. 2012; Szabat 2020; Wilkinson et al. 2014). Therefore, HCPs' are required to make an effort to avoid causing any unnecessary harm. Moreover, and according to the principle of benevolence HCPs are supposed to give parents and of ill children as well as patients and their loved ones hope or at least not take it away from them. Hope can help patients and parents cope with new challenges and avoid fear and despair (Bally et al. 2014, pp. 364–369). In addition, it is possible that HCPs can positively affect patients' hope by using strategies such as giving patients support through the PC values mentioned above such as psychological, physical and spiritual support (Mok 2010, pp. 877–883). The positive effects of patient-caregiver communication make it possible to build trust and confidence on both sides (Reinke 2010, pp. 985–988). Thus, maintaining hope in patients is an essential aspect of patients' right to information regarding their medical care.

When it comes to why certain expressions and metaphors used by HCPs could be hurtful to parents of seriously ill children and why the terms listed at the beginning of this section could be treated as offensives four basic reasons can be identified. The first one is that these terms objectivize fetuses and children. Phrases such as a child "would be a vegetable," future children would be "waste of money/time/energy," "there is nothing we can do for him/her," or "you can have another one," reveal strong economic factors underpinning the present or future of any human being's life. As was mentioned above, patients cannot in terms of their illness and treatment be treated solely as clients or as a sort of source of economic goods, which makes them vulnerable.

That is why HCPs are trained to become compassionate instead of indifferent and purely profit-oriented. The second reason is that the fetuses and children referred to in the above phrases are presented as the real cause of evil and suffering in place of the disease itself, when the opposite is in fact the case—it not children with life-threatening illnesses that are the cause of a family's suffering, but simply the illness itself.

The third reason is that claiming that seriously ill children "would live a life of suffering," "would ruin (somebody's) marriage," "would ruin (somebody's) family," or that "this child will hurt you/your family/your children" convey sinister messages that are contradicted by research on this topic. Indeed, studies show that families can handle the task of caring for seriously ill children. Moreover, such care may even bring family members closer together (Janvier et al. 2012; Szabat 2020).

The fourth and final reason is that these problematic phrases are not good communication choices for HCPs when trying to keep parental hope alive and encourage parents to feel positive about their future. The use of such terms as "incompatible with life," claiming that children "would live a meaningless life," and that the illness is "life threatening," reflect a counselor's subjective vision of the parents' lives, which the latter may perceive as an act of discrimination. Furthermore, making such assumptions cannot be classified as any type of clinical practice in any form. Therefore, the use of such terms to describe a fetus and a child is not only inappropriate, but also conveys to parents a counselor's negative image of their future children and their possible life with them.

At the end of this section, it is worth mentioning that the authors of one study advise HCPs to avoid the term "lethal" and recommend "that counseling should focus on salient prognostic features" (Wilkinson et al. 2014, p. 306). The authors of this research claim that the use of term "lethal" in clinical communication in the context of informing parents about such autosomal trisomies such as Edwards syndrome (T18) and Patau syndrome (T13) cannot be seen as a part of good clinical practice. The authors derive the word "lethal" from the Greek word "oblivion" referring to its personification—Lethe—daughter of Eris in Greek mythology and to its meaning as Lethe—a river (Wilkinson et al. 2014, p. 306; Oxford English Dictionary 2021). The connotations of the adjective "lethal" could be negative because of its etymological connection with death, shadows, forgetting the world of living, futility, etc. Further, the authors underline the fact that the term "incompatible with life" when used in a counseling context has the same clinically-negative impact on parents' well-being (Wilkinson et al. 2014, p. 307). The improvement in achieving a clinically-neutral language could rely on finding an alternative terms to inform parents about such a diagnosis e.g. "life-limiting," "a poor prognosis," "potentially lethal," or "malformations"

(Wilkinson et al. 2014, p. 308). However, as the authors themselves realize, their proposed new terms may also raise doubts because of their own possibly negative associations. Taking into account all the above-mentioned suggestions, the best communication strategy should be a personal explanation of the diagnosis in the most neutral language possible as well as further steps in terms of possible treatment.

Following these recommendations, it can be argued that a possible change in terminology from a clinically-negative language to clinically-neutral language could spare parents any unnecessary harm arising from receiving improperly-handled information. It could likewise help parents focus on new challenges that would require restructuring life priorities and making existentially important decisions. Moreover, a clinically-neutral language would leave room for hope, which, as the research shows, has a supportive function and allows parents to deal with vulnerable circumstances.

Conclusions

At the communication level, the principle "do no harm" concerns the way in which HCPs convey information about a sensitive diagnosis. In this context a question may be raised as to whether it is possible to weigh the degree of harm caused by a wrong diagnosis on a single scale against the poor or inaccurate communication of a proper diagnosis. Probably the most common answer to this question would be negative regarding the physical and psychological consequences of a wrong diagnosis. However, even if the mode of communication is not as important as the prescribed treatment and therapy, it still plays an important role in the therapeutic process, influencing parents' well-being and their capacity to become autonomous actors responsible for their children and their own decisions and choices. On the one hand, from the perspective of HCPs the most important aspect of medical care is to ensure a proper diagnosis as a basis for further treatment. On the other hand, any unnecessary harm should be avoided in therapeutic relationships between HCPs and parents so that the latter and their close ones can focus on handling the diagnosis and concentrating all their efforts on planning care, especially in the case of serious illness, when their daily lives and activities will require restructuring. Hence, the most effective communication strategy when handling highly sensitive issues in PPC is one that is personally tailored to the needs of each parent and that focuses on informing them of the diagnosis using medical language that is as neutral and understandable as possible. In addition, information on further possible treatment should be given without using any unnecessary comments on the part of HCPs, and it should leave room for hope, which has a supportive function, enabling parents to deal with highly difficult decisions.

References

Askitopoulou H., Vgontzas A.N. 2018. The relevance of the Hippocratic Oath to the ethical and moral values of contemporary medicine. Part I: The Hippocratic Oath from antiquity to modern times. *European Spine Journal* 27: 1481–1490.

Baalen van C.N., Grypdonck M., Hecke van A., Verhaeghe S. 2016. Hope dies last… A qualitative study into the meaning of hope for people with cancer in the palliative phase. *European Journal of Cancer Care* 25: 570–579.

Bally J.M., Duggleby W., Holtslander L., Mpofu C., Spurr S., Thomas R., Wright K. 2014. Keeping hope possible: A grounded theory study of the hope experience of parental caregivers who have children in treatment for cancer. *Cancer Nursing* 37(5): 363–372.

Beauchamp T.L., Childress J.F. 2001. *Principles of Biomedical Ethics*. New York: Oxford University Press.

Berterö C., Vanhanen M., Appelin G. 2008. Receiving a diagnosis of inoperable lung cancer: Patients' perspectives of how it affects their life situation and quality of life. *Acta Oncologica* 47: 862–869.

Bluebond-Langner M. 2016. Keeping all options open: Parents' approaches to advance care planning. *Health Expectations* 20: 675–684.

Brown E.M., Thorn C., Cowell D. 2016. Compassionate extubation in the home: It takes a team. *Journal of Pain and Symptom Management* 51(2): 337–338.

Clayton J.M., Hancock K., Parker S., Butow Ph.N., Walder S., Carrick S., Currow D., Ghersi D., Glare P., Hagerty R., Olver I.N., Tattersall M.H.N. 2008. Sustaining hope when communicating with terminally ill patients and their families: A systematic review. *Psycho-Oncology* 17: 641–659.

Cruft R., Liao S., Renzo M. (eds.) 2015. *Philosophical Foundations of Human Rights*. Oxford: Oxford University Press.

Daneault S., Dion D., Sicotte C., Yelle L., Mongeau S., Lussier V., Coulombe M., Paillé P. 2010. Hope and noncurative chemotherapies: Which affects the other? *Journal of Clinical Oncology* 28(13): 2310–2313.

Daneault S., Lussier V., Mongeau S., Yelle L., Côté A., Sicotte C., Paillé P., Dion D., Coulombe M. 2016. Ultimate journey of the terminally ill. Ways and pathways of hope. *Canadian Family Physician/Le Médecin de famille canadien* 62: 648–656.

Dufault K., Martocchio B.C. 1985. Symposium on compassionate care and the dying experience. Hope: Its spheres and dimensions. *Nursing Clinics of North America* 20(2): 379–391.

Duggleby W., Hicks D., Nekolaichuk C., Holtslander L., Williams A., Chambers Th., Eby J. 2012. Hope, older adults, and chronic illness: A metasynthesis of qualitative research. *Journal of Advanced Nursing* 68(6): 1211–1223.

Dworkin G. 1988. *The Theory and Practice of Autonomy*. Cambridge: Cambridge University Press.

Eliott J.A., Olver I.N. 2009. Hope, life, and death: A qualitative analysis of dying cancer patients' talk about hope. *Death Studies* 33: 609–638.

Feudtner C., Carroll K.W., Hexem K.R., Silberman J., Kang T.I., Kazak A.E. 2010. Parental hopeful patterns of thinking, emotions, and pediatric palliative care decision making a prospective cohort study. *Archives of Pediatrics and Adolescent Medicine* 164 (9): 831–839.

Friedrichsdorf S.J., Bruera E. 2018. Delivering pediatric palliative care: from denial, palliphobia, pallilalia to palliactive. *Children. Special issue of Pediatric Palliative Care* 5(9): 120.

Griffin J. 2008. *On Human Rights*. Oxford: Oxford University Press.

Griffin J. 2015. *What Can Philosophy Contribute to Ethics*. Oxford: Oxford University Press.

Hasson-Ohayon I., Galinsky D. 2009. Religiosity and hope: A path for women coping with a diagnosis of breast cancer. *Psychosomatics* 50: 525–533.

Heyland D.K., Barwich D., Pichora D., Dodek P., Lamontagne F., You J.J., Tayler C., Porterfield P., Sinuff T., Simon J. 2013. Failure to engage hospitalized elderly patients and their families in advance care planning. *JAMA Internal Medicine* 173(9): 778–787.

Innes S., Payne S. 2009. Advanced cancer patients' prognostic information preferences: A review. *Palliative Medicine* 23: 29–39.

Janvier A., Farlow B., Wilfond B.S. 2012. The experience of families with children with Trisomy 13 and 18 in social networks. *Pediatrics* 130(2): 293–298.

Kim S.Y., Kim J.M., Kim S.W., Kang H.J., Shin I.S., Shim H.J., Cho S.H., Chung I.J., Yoon J.S. 2014. Determinants of a hopeful attitude among family caregivers in a palliative care setting. *General Hospital Psychiatry* 36 (2): 165–171.

Mackenzie C., Stoljar N. (ed.) 2000. *Relational Autonomy: Feminist Perspectives on Autonomy, Agency, and the Social Self*. Oxford: Oxford University Press.

McClement S.E., Chochinov H.M. 2008. Hope in advanced cancer patients. *European Journal of Cancer* 44: 1169–1174.

Miyashita M., Morita T,, Sato K., Hirai K., Shima Y., Uchitomi Y. 2008. Good death inventory: A measure for evaluating good death from the bereaved family member's perspective. *Journal of Pain and Symptom Management* 35(5): 486–498.

Mok E., Lau K., Lam W., Chan L., Ng J., Chan K. 2010. Health-care professionals' perspective on hope in the palliative care setting. *Journal of Palliative Medicine* 13(7): 877–883.

Nickel J.W. 2007. *Making Sense of Human Rights*. 2nd ed. Oxford: Blackwell Publishing.

Olsman E., Leget C., Onwuteaka-Philipsen B., Willems D. 2014. Should palliative care patients' hope be truthful, helpful or valuable? An interpretative synthesis of literature describing healthcare professionals' perspectives on hope of palliative care patients. *Palliative Medicine* 28(1): 59–70.

Oxford English Dictionary online. 2021. Oxford University Press. Available at: https://www.oed.com/view/Entry/107522. Accessed: 20.03.2021.

Pellegrino E. D.1994. Patient and physician autonomy: Conflicting rights and obligations in the physician-patient relationship. *Journal of Contemporary Health Law & Policy* 10(1): 47–68.

Reinke L.F., Shannon S.E., Engelberg R.A., Young J.P., Curtis R.J. 2010. Supporting hope and prognostic information: nurses' perspectives on their role when patients have life-limiting prognoses. *Journal of Pain and Symptom Management* 39(6): 982–992.

Robinson C.A. 2012. "Our best hope is a cure." Hope in the context of advance care planning. *Palliative and Supportive Care* 10: 75–82.

Rumpold T., Schur S., Amering M., Ebert-Vogel A., Kirchheiner K., Masel E., Watzke H., Schrank B. 2017. Hope as determinant for psychiatric morbidity in family caregivers of advanced cancer patients. *Psycho-Oncology* 26 (5): 672–678.

Saunders C., Baines M., Dunlop R. 1995. *Living with Dying. A Guide to Palliative Care*. Oxford: Oxford University Press.

Saunders C. 2006. *Selected Writings 1958–2004*. Oxford–New York: Oxford University Press.

Shirado A., Morita T., Akazawa T., Miyashita M., Sato K., Tsuneto S., Shima Y. 2013. Both maintaining hope and preparing for death: Effects of physicians' and nurses' behaviors from bereaved family members' perspectives. *Journal of Pain and Symptom Management* 45(5): 848–858.

Stans S.E.A., Dalemans R.J.P., Roentgen U.R., Smeets H.W.H., Beurskens A.J.H.M. Who said dialogue conversations are easy? The communication between communication vulnerable people and health-care professionals: A qualitative study. *Health Expectations* 21(5): 848–857.

Szabat M. 2020. Parental experience of hope in pediatric palliative care: Critical reflections on an exemplar of parents of a child with Trisomy 18, *Nursing Inquiry* 27: e12341.

Vachon M., Fillion L., Achille M. 2009. A conceptual analysis of spirituality at the end of life. *Journal of Palliative Medicine* 12(1): 53–59.

Vliet L. van, Francke A., Tomson S., Plum N., Wall E. van der, Bensing J. 2013. When cure is no option: How explicit and hopeful can information be given? A qualitative study in breast cancer. *Patient Education and Counseling* 90: 315–322.

Walker P., Lovat T. 2015. Concepts of personhood and autonomy as they apply to end-of-life decisions in intensive care. *Medicine Health Care and Philosophy* 18(3): 309–315.

Wilkinson D., Crespigny de L., Xafis V. 2014. Ethical language and decision-making for prenatally diagnosed lethal malformations. *Seminars in Fetal and Neonatal Medicine* 19: 306–311.

Paulina Hornik

The Role and Importance of Family Support in Oncological or Long-Term Illness

Abstract

This article discusses the importance and function of family support for people suffering from oncological or long-term illness. It will also outline the difficulties such support may encounter. An analysis of the issues shows that from the first moment that illness is suspected and the patient undergoes tests right through to the final diagnosis, the patient experiences a constant sense of uncertainty regarding their health and prognosis, which is a cause of considerable emotional tension. The prospect of a serious, chronic, or life-threatening illness raises many difficult questions to which there is usually no simple answer. Finding themselves in an entirely new situation such a person is forced to reflect on their existence, make changes to their hitherto lifestyle, accept many limitations and restrictions and focus their thoughts on their disease. In these circumstances, social support, and especially the support of one's close family, takes on a special importance. Family support plays an extremely important role when the ill patient is a child. The natural environment for a child is the family home. As a consequence, there is no doubt that home care is the best form of care for children with terminal diseases during those times when they are not undergoing hospital treatment.

Keywords: family support, social support, long-term disease, life-threatening illness

Introduction

The family plays a fundamental and decisive role in the life of every human being. A healthy, loving, strong and united family is not only a point of reference, but also a vital anchor for its members. This becomes extremely important when someone falls ill. This paper discusses the importance and function of family support for a person affected by oncological or long-term disease. It will also outline the difficulties this type of support may cause.

The belief that the benevolent presence of other people has a beneficial effect on the health and well-being of an individual appears to be gaining traction in social consciousness. One of the most important forms of social support a cancer patient can receive is the care provided by their own family—this is emotional and evaluative support, which allows the patient to feel that they are still loved, needed, important and accepted, no matter what happens next, no matter what they will look like, how they will behave, even if they lose control over their physical and mental functions. Regardless of all these things, the ill individual wants to feel and hear the words: I will be with you, I will not leave you, you will not be left alone (Baczewska et al. 2015, p. 46).

Family support

People need the support of other people, especially when they have exhausted their own ways of dealing with the problem. They feel helpless and fear losing control over their lives. Psycho-oncologists believe that such support depends on the ability to listen, and it exists when a person feels that someone understands and respects their fears. Research clearly indicates that expressing feelings related to problems or traumatic challenges reduces physiological arousal and mental stress. It is important to open up to someone you can trust rather than accept advice. Thanks to such support, the patient has the opportunity to overcome their own problems, difficulties, conflicts or complicated situations. This specific form of help assumes that those providing the support reinforce the recipients' strength and will to independently overcome obstacles.

Psychological support has an extremely positive impact on physical and mental health. In everyday life, everyone needs support, but in the face of illness it becomes even more essential. The essence of intelligently provided support lies in adjusting interactions to human needs at various stages of the illness. An analysis of these issues shows that, from the moment the illness is first suspected right through to the conducting of tests and the final diagnosis, the patient experiences constant uncertainty regarding their health and future prognosis, which is a source of considerable anxiety. The prospect of a serious, chronic, life-threatening disease gives rise to many difficult questions to which there is usually no simple answer.

Such a situation triggers many different emotions and forms of behavior in patients, which to external observers may seem incomprehensible or even exaggerated, e.g. anger, aggression, regret, despair, black eyes, incomprehension, loneliness, withdrawal, anxiety, depression and even suicide attempts. The new situation such a person finds themselves in forces them to reflect on their existence, make changes in their hitherto lifestyle, accept many limitations and focus their attention on the disease itself. Sometimes the emotional shock accompanying a diagnosis of cancer causes the patient to experience the unreality of their situation. In these circumstances, social support, and especially the support of the patient's closest family members, takes on a special importance (Parzyszek and Samorańska 2017, p. 9).

Family support plays an extremely important role when the ill person is a child. The natural environment for a child is the family home. As a consequence, home care is undoubtedly the best form of care for children suffering from a terminal illness during those times they are not undergoing hospital treatment.

A child's suffering and illness constitute a special situation in which family support clearly plays an irreplaceable and invaluable role. A child with a long-term or high-risk illness can affect the quality of family ties in various ways—it can strengthen, strain or destroy them. A child is like a sensitive seismograph, picking up any subtle changes in the relationships between his relatives taking place in the background of his illness. The unconditional love that an ill child receives from his immediate family is invaluable. The task of parents and the immediate family, in particular, is to show support for the child in a constructive way. It takes a considerable amount of love that is expressed wisely. When considering the methods of such support, attention should be paid to such areas of family functioning as being and acting (Gątarek 2017, p. 160).

The ability of parents to adjust to the situation in constructive ways constitutes the final phase in the adaptation to the child's illness. This process begins when the disease is diagnosed. The initial shock and numbness is followed by an emotional crisis. Parents are confronted with questions asked by their child that cannot be answered by anyone. It is also often the case that they blame themselves, feel remorse, and irrational guilt that somehow they could have prevented the disease. Gradually, they slowly begin to adapt to the situation, but this is only a phase in adapting to an illusion. Subconsciously, within the panorama of inner feelings, rebellion and a refusal to consent to the situation. There are no rigidly defined timeframes for the duration of individual stages of this process, but usually it is long-lasting. The final stage in this difficult journey in overcoming subsequent phases of adaptation to the child's illness is constructive adaptation, which results in a loving presence and thoughtful action (Gątarek 2017, p. 160).

A chronic disease or a disease with an unfavorable life-threatening diagnosis, not only disturbs the physical functioning of the child, but also its psychosocial functioning (in the social, personality and family sphere). It should be borne in mind that the needs of chronically ill children are not only biological needs, but, most of all, the need for security, belonging, contact with other people, the need for self-acceptance, the need for acceptance and love from others (especially in the family environment), and, finally, the need for action and self-realization, which adults often forget when losing a child. A strong family with consistent inner values creates a climate of security for a child and can become a buffer against the changes taking place in a reality marred by illness (Gątarek 2017, p. 160).

We can define the family as an interpersonal social system, which is also a kind of social institution. In it, the child learns to adopt attitudes towards the mysteries of life, death, health and disease. When a child is ill, his relative face difficult challenges, which become determinants of the further functioning of the family. It happens that one of these challengers is the need to confront inevitable death (Wojciechowski 2017, p. 217).

The natural environment for a child is the family home. As such, there is no doubt that home care is the best form of care for a child with life-limiting conditions when not undergoing hospital treatment. Children at home, using medical devices, surrounded by the love and care of their relatives, more quickly accept the technology that has become part of their lives. For example, children with respiratory failure included in the home mechanical ventilation program do not treat the ventilator as an "enemy" but rather as something that helps them breathe (Pokusa-Baran et al. 2015, p. 257). The Home Hospice of Mary Queen of the Apostles in Kraków illustrates this fact well. From the various, long-term observations of the Hospice's team, it can be concluded that the family members of the patient who know the prognosis and know that there is little time left for them all to be together, to forgive each other, and to deepen their relationship, most often mobilize themselves, and the ill person can experience a lot of good and feel the engagement of their family, who can meet their needs. For example, there are cases where relatives of the patient return from abroad to be with the patient, who eagerly awaits them. One of the hospice's wards was in agony for three days. On the morning of the third day, when her sister, whom she had not seen for many years, came from abroad, she got up and for a week she ate normally, drank, talked, and enjoyed the presence of her sibling. A week later she died. The family is thus very important to the patient, especially in the terminal stage of illness. Patients are happier when they have a loved one with them.

Sometimes a patient leaves a hospital in poor health and is taken into hospice care. If they are straight from the hospital straight to an inpatient hospice, they will probably remain in the same state, while when they are returned to their homes, their condition remains stable due to a better quality of life and the presence of relatives. Hence, when an ill person is provided with appropriate medical care at home, an ill person can live longer. Ill people stay with their relatives until the very end. However, health conditions do not always allow an ill person to stay at home, even if the family would very much like for this to be the case.

The role of family support for people suffering from cancer

The role of family support for a cancer patient was discussed in the article entitled "Being cared by a family member: The existential feelings of cancer patients." The study involved 20 patients treated in primary health care facilities in Northeast Parana, Brazil. The data was collected primarily on the basis of the following research question: "What has been your experience of being cared for by your family?" (Wakiuchi et al. 2015, p. 381).

Based on the findings of this study, it can be concluded that the severity of a cancer prognosis is usually associated with fear and negative associations that affect different spheres of life, especially quality of life after the commencement of treatment. Hence, as experiences related to the everyday life of people with cancer are inscribed in a wider social context, so both patients and their families experience uncertainty and feel insecure. Given the relationship between cancer, suffering and deterioration, it becomes clear that the patient and his family must confront problems that go far beyond the mere physical manifestations of the disease. It requires understanding and emotional support from family members in accordance with the patient's needs at a given stage of experiencing the disease. To meet these needs, the authors of this article urge that palliative care should be introduced at the time of the cancer diagnosis as it enables patients and their families to actively participate in the therapeutic process, to make decisions together and to act as a team in the face of treatment and care options. Furthermore, the everyday life of patients and their caregivers who are also members of their family is based an extremely close relationship that can both strengthen bonds and reciprocity, but also trigger conflicts and misunderstandings expressed via various emotions. It is doubly difficult because cancer patients experience both their own emotions related to the disease and treatment, as well as specific feelings and anxieties that permeate the family environment in which they receive their care and treatment. If the patient feels genuine commitment and attention from family members they are less likely to feel addicted or the object of onerous duties for others, and this is conducive to the constructive resolution of any problems that may arise during the care process. Total suffering that embraces all dimensions of human existence, especially if it is a long-term process, is a challenge not only for a person marked by the stigma of pain and disease, but also, albeit somewhat differently, for their environment. In their analysis of interviews with ill people, the authors sometimes noticed that family members provide care, but at the same time maintain a certain internal distance from the caregiver. In such a scenario the caregivers are with the ill, but are not open to being with them, which requires inner engagement, closeness and empathy (Wakiuchi et al. 2015, pp. 383–388).

The authors reported that the patients experienced in their discourse a certain "affective detachment" from their families. In other words, their family members were physically close to them, but at the same time were emotionally distant, because they did not participate in their suffering. The desire to know what the ill person felt was limited only to superficial perceptions and avoiding being truly open to the idea of exposing themselves to what the patient was actually experiencing. By running away from what is unpleasant, family members then deprive themselves of the possibility of being with the patient in any authentic way. In addition, despite the lack of emotional involvement of other family members, even in the face of difficulties in cancer treatment, ill people remain the mainstay of support in their homes. By crossing the barriers imposed by the disease, patients try to care for others ill (Wakiuchi et al. 2015, pp. 384–385).

The experiences of other patients show how loving care can pave the way for others to take responsibility. In other words—genuine care gives the patient the opportunity to be themselves. Caring for a family member with cancer through genuine manifestations of care allows caregivers to enter the existential dimension of the patient. Such care takes the form of "being-with-the-other." From the moment the family recognizes itself as the center of care and takes full responsibility for this task, the process of positively influencing the patient's coping strategy, decision making, daily self-care and showing affection begins. Even patients who did not explicitly express their feelings of gratitude recognized the importance of a family that was actively present and found it of great value (Wakiuchi et al. 2015, pp. 385–386). Participants' statements show that the unconditional support of families caring for the health and the well-being of patients was reflected in the latter's feelings. For these patients, the care they received exceeded expectations and they did not feel neglected. When proper care was provided and family relationships were valued, patients did not report moments of loneliness or suffering. Moreover, they defined the healing period as a time when the patient experienced unity with the family, sharing and love. This is where family members take a leading role in overcoming the obstacles associated with cancer and, in addition, by reorganizing all home dynamics to adapt to the new conditions imposed by the disease, they become the most important pillar of psychological support.

Caring for a family member suffering from cancer through genuine manifestations of care allows caregivers to enter the patient's existential dimension. Family members communicate in a shared world of coexistence where they are, and always have been, available to others. A total commitment to others, most often manifested in small gestures, seems to reduce the burden of cancer and the suffering that comes with it, as this burden is ultimately shared between the ill person and the caregiver. Such ties between the patient and the caregiver exude feelings of great joy and gratitude, which was reflected in the faces of the interviewees when they refer to the person who is caring for them. According to what the patients said, the care they received could overcome the torment of cancer and made this difficult experience an opportunity for others to demonstrate unconditional care and presence in their lives (Wakiuchi et al. 2015, pp. 386–387).

Despite a cultural heritage that sees women as primary caregivers, the authors of this article have found that the interviewed patients were looked after by both men and women. In the case of married couples, spouses remained faithful to each other, and the-care they provided their ill loved ones gave a new a lease of life to the feelings between them. Their statements show how illness restored the relationship between husband and wife. The difficulties of living with cancer revived the realm of feelings, and these were reflected in kindness, affection and dedication to others. Effective family care depends on the existence of positive, deep relationships. When caring is intertwined with love, affection, and kindness, the attitudes and feelings that are associated with engagement in another human being are rooted in real desire, thereby making such emptions truly authentic. When caring is a consequence of love, it happens naturally. Thus, to sum up, those patients who received genuine care from their families reported that this had a positive influence on the course of their illness and their lives. Amidst the difficulties caused by illness, they found an opportunity for their own development, thanks to the care they received from their families. Their life took on a new meaning thanks to the establishment of stronger bonds and a sense of appreciation and gratitude for the attitudes of their carers (Wakiuchi et al. 2015, p. 387).

Conclusions

Family support for a patient is rooted in interpersonal resources, and protects against the negative effects of stress by satisfying the needs that arise during the illness. A lack of support from friends and loved ones has certain consequences. It engenders feelings of loneliness and isolation and increases anxiety. In addition, a lack of support can even lead to depression and an increased sense of loneliness. This may be accompanied by a sense of hopelessness and helplessness, a lack of joy in life, and a belief in one's own worthlessness. If this perception of a lack of support and the loneliness it entails become permanent experiences, it may lead to the disintegration of the personality, which most often also affects the patient's physical condition.

Doctors often emphasize the fact that a patient who is supported by their family goes through the treatment process with much better effects. The patient responds more positively to treatment and sometimes even recovers—this phenomenon applies to both physical and mental reactions. The body copes better with pain, and repair and regenerative mechanisms are more effective when the patient has "something to live for." Zbigniew Pawlak reminds us that

> in order to understand how important it is for an ill person in their suffering and dying to be self-sacrificing, it is necessary to realize that an ill person can endure a great deal, provided that they are not abandoned and left alone. In loneliness, the spiraling effects of pain and fear eventually reach a point of despair and madness [...], being simply present with an ill person is the first treatment, and it is strictly medical and sanitary treatment (Pawlak 2000).

Similarly in the book *Live until the End. A Disease Manual*, one of the most important messages is a call to cultivate closeness in our relationships. During a conversation with Katarzyna Jabłońska, Jan Kaczkowski says that "In life in general, that is also in life with illness, the most important thing is closeness. A person who has experienced closeness has a better life" (Kaczkowski 2018).

For patients, the problems caused by their illness are not obstacles to self-development, when they feel they have support from their relatives. They find an opportunity for development. Their lives take on a new meaning thanks to the deepening of these bonds and a sense of appreciation and gratitude for the attitudes of those who provide them with care, time, empathy, and genuine presence. The existence of a good, deep relationship is essential to effective family care. Saint Augustine said that "Where there is love there is no suffering and even if it is, it becomes the same object of love" (Saint Augustine) When caring is-complemented with love, affection, and kindness, commitment and attention come from an authentic desire. When caring is a consequence of love, it happens naturally.

References

Baczewska B., Binnebesel J., Block LB., Glaza M., Kulik A., Musiał D., Rydz E., Stelcer B., Wojciechowska K. 2015. Pomiędzy życiem a nieżyciem. Psychologiczna analiza dynamiki egzystencjalnej w przebiegu choroby nowotworowej. In *W drodze do brzegu życia*, eds. E. Krajewska, C.R, Łukaszuk, J. Lewko, W. Kułak, 35–75. Białystok: Uniwersytet Medyczny w Białymstoku.

Gątarek I. 2017. Środowisko rodzinne a doświadczanie choroby przewlekłej dziecka – konteksty opieki i edukacji. In *Rodzina – wsparcie i pomoc*, eds. M. Parzyszek, M. Samorańska, 151–164. Lublin: Episteme.

Kaczkowski J. 2018. Ksiądz Jan Kaczkowski i spokój umierania. *Więź*. Available at: http://wiez.com.pl/2018/02/09/ks-jan-kaczkowski-i-spokoj-umierania/ Accessed: 13.09.2020.

Parzyszek M., Samorańska M. (eds.) 2017. *Rodzina – wsparcie i pomoc*. Lublin: Episteme.

Pawlak Z. 2000. Opieka duchowa w terminalnej fazie choroby. *Nowa Medycyna* 1. Czytelnia Medyczna BORGIS. Accessed: 13.09.2020.

Pokusa-Baran A., Kulik H., Dobrzyń-Matusiak D. 2015. Funkcjonowanie i rola rodziny w opiece nad dzieckiem wentylowanym mechanicznie metodą inwazyjną w warunkach domowych. In *W drodze do brzegu życia*, eds. E. Krajewska, C.R. Łukaszuk, J. Lewko, W. Kułak, 256–270. Białystok: Uniwersytet Medyczny w Białymstoku.

Saint Augustine. Available at: https://www.augustianie.pl/sw-augustyn-2/sw-augustyn-mysli/ Accessed: 17.10.2020.

Wakiuchi J., Oliveira Salimena A.M. de, Aparecida Sales C. 2015. Being cared by a family member: The existential feelings of cancer patients. *Text Context Nursing* 24(2): 381–389.

Wojciechowski F. 2017. *Niepełnosprawność. Rodzina. Dorastanie*. Warszawa: Żak.

Anthropology and Philosophy of Death and Dying

Anna E. Kubiak

End-of-Life Issues in the Context of Biopolitics and Bioeconomy*

Abstract

End-of-life issues such as the question of the border between life and death, controversies around bioeconomization of the human body and commodification of life, around the ethical dimensions of terminating one's life and the consequences of legalization of assisted death are more and more objects of public and expert debate. There are broader reasons for this: the advance of medical technology, hybridization of living forms, posthumanist reflection, bioart, the unprecedented scale of ageing of the human population and the consequences of this process expressed in an apocalyptic tone, and the vision of the extinction of *homo sapiens* thanks to climate change. Doubt in the omnipotent knowledge of experts, pluralisation of social norms, blurring of the borders of crucial categories, social movements that resist biopolitical and bioeconomic powers are shaking the foundations of biopolitics. Despite mobilization of biopolitics and the growing expansion of the bioeconomy I will give examples of "junction points" which are mediation-resistant, driving biopolitics into "implosion" (in Baudrillard's sense).

Keywords: end-of-life, death, bioeconomy, biopolitics, bare life, aging

Introduction: Death is not taboo any more

End-of-life issues, such as the question of the border between life and death, controversies around commercialization of the human body, and the ethical

---

* This chapter comes from the book: Kubiak 2020. Published with the permission of Cambridge Scholars Publishing.

dimensions of terminating one's life are more and more objects of public and expert debate. Debates on legalization of assisted death—euthanasia and physician assisted suicide—arise in Europe, America, Australia and in many other places. Death is not taboo any more. The consciousness about death as a personal and global issue is growing. There are more and more voices saying that we are living in the shadow of a volcano—an ecological catastrophe.

Death is a definite end of life in the individual form. Despite medicalization of death, despite debating about end-of-life issues in the context of the medical definitions of death, law, economy, life sciences' technologies, and abstract, universalized values in bioethical theories, death is also something different. Bioethics and law focuses on the question, what is to be done, which options for decision-making are? All these disciplines reduce life to "bare life" (in Agamben's sense). Thus, they fail to account for the ontological, psychological, relational, personal, and spiritual (even in an atheistic worldview) event and process of dying. I will shortly remind theories of biopolitics, bioeconomy and bare life. Theorizing about death we cannot escape the issue of life, be it an opposition or continuity of death.

Biopolitics

Foucault traces the history of power by drawing on the development from disciplinary society to biopolitics. When considering power over life and death in the age of the disciplinary society, Foucault argues that this relied on the ability to condemn to death and to allow living: "The right which was formulated as the 'power of life and death' was in reality the right to *take* life or *let* live" (Foucault 2013, p. 42). He demonstrates the process of transferring the technology of power from the sovereign, who has the right to leave alive and sentence to death, to the biopolitics, forcing upon life the power of sentencing to life and allowing to die. Modern life administrators are concerned with "a bare issue of surviving" at the level of the whole population (Foucault 2010, p. 94). In other words: "the ancient right to take life or let live was replaced by a power to *foster* life or *disallow* it to the point of death" (Foucault 2013, p. 43).

Biopolitics is focused on body and on the processes of life and its main goal is investing in life. It does not eliminate but completes the old disciplinary techniques of power, working on different level. Disciplinary society operates on individual bodies, whereas biopolitics on the level of population. Jean Baudrillard highlights the politicization of the biological meaning of life and death and the biopolitics of controlling it. He emphasizes the archetypal meaning of the border between life and death in a symbolic exchange, and its monopolization by power. Thus, biopolitics, by controlling life also monopolizes death. Power, located in the gap between the subject and his/her body (Baudrillard 2007, p. 163), rationalizes life and death:

> no one may freely dispose of one's own life and death; each of us must get social approval. It cannot even be allowed that life and death depend on biological accident, since a certain amount of freedom would still be concealed. Our basic moral imperative is therefore not only 'do not kill' but also 'do not die'—in any case not in any way you can freely choose—you can die only under the condition that the law, supported by medicine, authorizes (Baudrillard 2007, pp. 225–226).

In the 21st century the characteristic process of postponing the private moment of death by excessive medicalization and bureaucratization in the last stages of the trajectory of the dying person continues. The right to live is strictly related to the ban on dying and the obligation to care about a biological body, the *corpus*. Life and death became a political object in the hands of medical and legislative mechanisms, which control, monitor, and organize collective vitality, morbidity, and mortality.

Bioeconomy

The notion of "bioeconomy" was first used in an OECD (the Organization for Economic Cooperation and Development) report, "capturing the sense that contemporary capitalism is increasingly based on the capacity to in various ways explore and commercially exploit biological resources" (Styhre 2012, p. 190). The term denotes "the intersection of, and mutual dependence on, economic activities and the life sciences" (Styhre 2012, p. 416). The concept of bioeconomy was developed by Nikolas Rose (2007). According to Rose, after the politics of health and demographics in the 18th and 19th centuries a shift occurred so that we now have politics "concerned with our growing capacities to control, manage, engineer, reshape, and modulate the very vital capacities of human beings as living creatures. It is, I suggest, a politics of life itself" (Rose 2007, p. 3).

Bioeconomy has a transnational character in a globalized world. It operates on a trans-individual level in a global market of blood, embryos, sperm, cells, etc. "The biological entities that inhabit this landscape (the economic enterprises—AEK) are no longer just individuals and populations—the twin poles of Foucault's biopower—but also cells, molecules, genomes, and genes" (Helmreich 2008, p. 461). It is important to note the word "also," because analogously, like Foucault's contention that biopolitics does not exclude disciplinary power, it is the same with bioeconomy. Bioeconomy is an additional and different level of power in late-modern society. While biopolitics characterized the modernity of the 19th century and first half of the 20th century, bioeconomy, starting from the second half of the 20th century (the end of the 1970s with the development of neoliberal doctrines), is characteristic of 21st century power relations. The norm of improving life and health acquires new meaning: the accumulation of capital. As Styhre notices: "The neoliberal doctrine has helped both to justify the treatment of biological assets in economic terms and to provide the tools and theories for translating these assets into financial terms" (Styhre 2012, p. 1377).

Bioeconomy applies to transfers between different bodies (transplantation between bodies and technologies: chip implantation, artificial organs). Human material transcends the living man, in that it (human material) can become part of a bank (e.g., of blood), information (in databases), semen, or an animal kept as a stem cell (Lemke 2010, pp. 109–110). Bioeconomy strengthens the social norms concentrated on "bare life," as the perfect (in esthetic categories) and healthy body becomes the most desired commodity. "Bare life" acquires economic, surplus value.

Bare life

In contrast to Foucault, Giorgio Agamben finds the ancient roots of biopolitics, and considers it through the optics of the political structure of the "state of emergency" and, its extreme form, the concentration camp. Where Foucault saw population in the foundation of biopolitics, Agamben sees "bare life," *homo sacer*, the patient in *coma depassé*, and *Muselmann*, as the center in which biopower operates. He considers biopolitics to be the root of Western political activity both in liberal democracies and in totalitarian systems. The philosopher refers to Aristotelian notions of *zoe* and *bios*. In ancient Greece *zoe* was a life as such and belonged to *oikos*, private life, whereas *bios* was a good life and belonged to *polis*, a public life. Biopolitics of modern Western societies is directed at exposed "bare life" which is a new constellation of *zoe* and *bios*. *Zoe* is equated with anonymous, biological life, as opposed to *bios*, which is civil life (Agamben 2008a, p. 170). He develops this thought: "bare life" is a border line sphere of non-distinguishability between *bios* and *zoe* (Agamben 2008a, p. 20), thus *bios* disappears. Nowadays it is biological life which is the center of political life. The implications are as follows: "bare life" is connected with law in ways which exclude a discourse about life outside legal order; there is no return to the category of *bios* as a political life, and "bare life" becomes the hidden fundament of Western political orders.

Referring to contemporary debates on euthanasia (after discussion of the eugenics of Nazi Germany), Agamben focuses on extreme cases such as *coma dépassé* or brain death, in which a person is unable to express his or her will (Agamben 2008a, pp. 219–226). Decisions concerning these beings situated in a "zone of uncertainty" (Agamben 2008a, p. 224) between life and death, seem obvious examples of how "life" and "death" become "political concepts, which, as such, take on exact meaning only by a decision" (Agamben 2008a, p. 225). The philosopher states emphatically: "the biological fact is in itself immediately political and *vice versa*" (Agamben 2008a, p. 201). The arbitrary decision which life is worth and which is unworthy to live is important because of the possibility of transplantation. The new entities, named by Willard Gaylin (1974) "neomortos," persons in a vegetative state, occupy an indeterminate zone between life and death. They represent the extreme example of "bare life" that is at stake in the biopolitical game. He completes Foucault's formula for biopolitics ("the right to make live and to let die") in this way: "to sentence to outlive" (Agamben 2008b, p. 156).

Conclusions of this part of the paper

We live in a culture in which medical and legal authorities and practices encircle our life and death. Life—in the meaning of "bare life"—has been politicized and economized, and a body is treated as impersonal object, in transplantation practice—transpersonal complex of exchangeable body parts. The meaning of life and death is changing as part of the processes of biocapitalization and biomedicalization. Life and death in the age of bioeconomy are not natural categories. They are "naturalized" (in the sense of Roland Barthes) in ideologies and strategies of biopolitics. Life is being reinvented by the life sciences collaborating with the global market and became a commodity. The neoliberal regime treats biological assets as biocapital. The meaning of life has been reframed while becoming part of the capitalist process of accumulation.

Patients act according to rules of biopolitics and have become consumers, demanding that their problems be resolved by drugs or treatment. Both—pro-life and pro-choice ("my body, my choice") discourses are inscribing themselves in biopolitical strategies: both defend the concept of "bare life," in terms of "sacred life" (but in practice biological life)—in case of pro-life camp—or in categories of life which is worth or which is unworthy to live—in case of pro-choice camp. Thus, a discourse for or against assisted dying does not have to mean a decision for or against biopolitics. It should be pointed out that the discourse for and against assisted dying corresponds to a high status attributed to the body. After all, people ask for assisted dying because of a loss of proper health.

The neoliberal ethos encourages decision-making about the time and conditions of dying (congruent with the idea of man as an entrepreneur in all facets of life), but these decisions must be subjected to examination by legal and medical authorities and institutions. In accordance with the model of *homo economicus* and the consumer, one might expect new treatments such as euthanasia. Conceiving oneself as human capital, one calculates the costs of one's living, dying, medical treatment, and the welfare of one's family.

Shaking the foundations of biopolitics

In this part I will analyse different areas of biopolitics and bioeconomy in order to display "folds," tiny "cracks" in the foundations of biopower. I argue that biopolitics has gradually descended into crisis since the end of the 1960s when the debates on the definition of death started. The outcome of this quiet evolution (rather than revolution) is unknown but is expressed in a blurring of the borders of the crucial categories, first of all between life and death, but also between human beings and animals, human beings and cyborgs, culture and nature, along with anomalies questioning paradigms of the regimes of truth. I do not suggest that the emancipation movement for "letting die" will be necessarily followed by the radical transgression of biopower. I only observe that there are growing margins, "grey zones," beyond the core of biopower, embodied in patient's groups fighting for their rights, individuals claiming the right to their death, and pro-euthanasia social movements, working for the legalisation of euthanasia and assisted suicide.

From the other side I observe that this is the reason why biopolitics is undergoing a mobilization in the form of proliferation of norms (e.g. legislative, medical), of more and more instruments applied: medical and bioethical commissions,[1] legislative interventions, churches' declarations against "death culture," social pro-life movements, the discourses of the "promissive potential"[2] (e.g., of life sciences, the pharmaceutical industry, shareholder value ideologies and travel agencies), and all projects for "making life." Junction

---

[1] E.g. the Presidential Council for Bioethics in 2001 in the United States (Sandel 2007).

[2] "Scientists aware of the public distrust, started to include in the production of knowledge the discourse of the promissive potential of the manipulation of biology, under the name of 'regenerative medicine'" (Franklin 2003).

points described in this part engage biopolitics in producing regulatory and repair mechanisms.

The area of uncertainty and unpredictability is driving biopolitics into a crisis. I use the notion of "uncertainty" to express the impression of being struck by anxiety, public distrust in a biotechnological revolution and the growing consciousness that fewer and fewer things depend on individual projects (in Giddens' sense) and this anxiety and distrust act in opposition to the ideology of neoliberalism. A spectra of ecological catastrophe and the threat of a definitive end of human civilization, a pandemic of corona virus disease (COVID-19), terrorism, global violence (Mbembe 2018), genocides, the tragedy on Utoha (Farrell 1998, p. 16), expressed in apocalyptic visions (e.g. Girard 2018) in popular culture, create situations where political and social control is weak and the only possible action is to try to lessen the negative consequences, to mobilize additional forces to build dams against a flood. Pandemic deepen this feeling of uncertainty. Living in border time we lost—as R.D. Laing and A. Giddens would say—ontological security. I see the split between late modernity with its immunological systems described by Ulrich Beck (2002) and Roberto Esposito (2015) and our crisis-time, when we still build security systems but do not believe in their perfect protection. As Kirby Farrell writes: "It reflects a disturbance in the ground of collective experience: a shock to people's values, trust, and sense of purpose; an obsessive awareness that nations, leaders, even we ourselves, can die" (Farrell 1998, p. 3).

The category of "uncertainty" which I use in describing medical, legislative and economic issues may be a key argument for the fact that biopower instruments face resistance. It is difficult to prognosticate a radical change in reaction to the main symptoms of our unstable time but if there is one, it will not be a revolution or an explosion but rather an "implosion." By this notion Baudrillard means a threat to accumulation, power and consumer society that can be "dismantled, but [implosion—AEK] does not stem from revolutionary resistance from outside, but from a kind of dissolution from inside" (Devisch and Hoyweghen 2011, p. 18). He defines "implosion" as:

> The absorption of one pole into another, the short circuiting between poles of every differential system of meaning, the erasure of distinct terms and oppositions, including that of the medium and of the real—thus the impossibility of any mediation, of any dialectical intervention between the two or from one to the other (Baudrillard 2001, p. 83).

Foucault notes that everywhere where power works there is "the strategic field of power relations" (Foucault 2010, p. 69) of resistance and it always operates inside a network of power. But—I assert—the ambiguity of the borders of basic categories such as culture/nature, life/death and economic *aporia* described below, is intensified in the 21st century and cannot be resolved on a practical level, inside a network of biopolitics and bioeconomy. Because the ground has started to exhibit its friable consistency, so the cracks have appeared in the foundations of institutions, social practices and discourses which are being problematised.

Ambiguity of the border between life and death

Despite mobilization of biopolitics and the growing expansion of the bioeconomy I will give examples of "junction points" which are mediation-resistant, driving biopolitics in crisis. By "junction points" I mean issues and fields where contradictions of ideas are not resolved, and where are different opinions and arguments on ethical, ontological, political economy and practical problems.

New, hard to classify beings, not showing the modern expectations of people as a self-reflection, are: brain-dead people, patients in a vegetative state, "locked in" patients, those with minimal consciousness, in a coma, cases of cerebral death, Alzheimer's patients, those with severe dementia, new-borns without a brain, those with a damaged autonomic nervous system, genetically modified animals, stem cells, embryos, hybrids/cyborgs (Lock 2003, p. 171). Hybridization is defined by Peter Stallybrass and Allon White as: "[a] mixing of binary opposites [...] such that there is a heterodox merging of elements usually perceived as incompatible which unsettles any fixed binaryism" (Stallybrass and White 1986, p. 44).

As authors of the book *Beyond the Body* write about such not-fully-alive or not-fully dead people, they are usually called "vegetables" and they are "hybrids in that they confuse the cultural categories of life and death; they represent the dissolution of Boundaries which organize key phases of the life course" (Hallam et al. 1999, p. 1).

Transgression of these limits—between life and death—is, in the current culture, associated with power and danger. There are in consequence conflicting diagnoses. Margaret Lock says that: "Among the thirty-two intensivists (specialists who work in ICUs) whom I interviewed between 1995 and 1997, not one believes that brain death signals the end of biological life [...]. As one intensivist put it, 'It is not death, but it is an irreversible diagnosis, which I accept'" (Lock 2003, pp. 171–172).

Defining a border between life and death is particularly difficult in the case of "those patients whose condition is 'masked' by the technology of intensive therapy units" (Evans 1994, p. 1), which are the best examples of cyborgs combining elements of human body and technology.

Uncertainty in life sciences and medical practices

The ambivalence of the status of hybrids causes hesitations during diagnosis. Theory has not completely been translated into practice. Dead person with a diagnosis according to brainstem death, may remain rosy, warm, and is even able to give birth to a child. The biggest challenges come from 21st century life sciences. Hogle focuses on tissue engineering and the commercialization of biological products. This field—the next step on from transplantation—produces hybrids of human tissue and synthetic materials. She observes that the life sciences bring confusion to our understanding of what is "normal." Biotechnology "produces a new imaginary about life" (Hogle 2003, p. 89) and death, and about the relation between nature and culture. Sarah Franklin refers to the issue of the capitalization of biology, using the example of cloning. The image of Dolly the sheep became the icon of genetic cloning, but also—in a social context—an omen of uncertainty and anxiety. In an age in which social consciousness is growing in relation to genetically modified products, pro-life movements are opposed to embryo research, and animal activists voice their objections to the instrumentalization of animals, bioscientists have started to develop strategies to cope with feelings of uncertainty. The new market in human tissue cloning is one example of the field of "biological control." According to Franklin the term means on the one hand rewriting life that "enables formerly 'absolute' biological boundaries to be crossed" (Franklin 2003, p. 101), and on the other, a tension between control and loss of control as the scientists themselves confess that they cannot predict all the effects of their practices.

From the point of view of Foucault's and Agamben's interpretation, we cannot speak about escaping biopolitics in any way other than by suicide. However, do not Foucault and Agamben, in sensitising to the issue related with bioauthority, take away these residues of subjectivity that have remained? Is a hybrid-body (connected to medical, technological instruments) still a "bare life"?

Many authors question the body as the essence of identity, proposing thinking rather about the multiplicity of a body or a "multispecies ecosystem" (Catts and Zurr 2016, p. 136) which is inhabited by a diversity of species, such as microbiomes. Such ecosystems are in constant differentiation. All these mutations are best described in the posthumanistic literature, in the paradigm of multiplication, the thing turn, and new materialism.

Aporia of economization of living and dying

Baudrillard indicates the contradiction of the political economy of death: from one side the institutional system "assigns excessive funds to prolong life as a value" (Baudrillard 2007, p. 225) but from the other side these choices of economic redistribution are dangerous for economic balance. So—according to the philosopher—euthanasia comes to the rescue to stabilize the nation's budget. He undermines the humanitarian aspect of assisted dying as "it perfectly matches the medium and long-term logics of the system itself. The aim in this case is empowering the social control" (Baudrillard 2007, p. 225).

With aging, growing morbidity of populations, the growing shortage of doctors and nurses, and the economic burden of hospitalization, home health care, pharmaceutics, physician services and medical technologies, there are dilemmas that are difficult to resolve. There is *aporia* between the absolute value of life and economic limitations, shaking the biopolitical regulations. There is contradiction in neoliberal ideology between narration about human rights and the actual situation. Here biopolitical mechanisms outlined by Agamben unfold: differentiation between life which is worth living and unworthy of being lived. As Spicker writes, we must "answer the question of how much ICU care should be provided to persons who not only could, but wish to, benefit from such treatment. Moreover, we shall have to reconsider where properly to draw the line concerning who is and who is not to receive ICU treatment" (Spicker 1996, p. 93).

Neoliberal political rationality aims to get rid of subjects it perceives to be burdensome. However, because neoliberalism demands its ethos be sustained through social norms and non-interference, it cannot overtly allow forms of killing. So it works in the way one could call covert non-voluntary euthanasia. It is evident in Poland that people die quicker because of waiting months or years for an operation or the proper rehabilitation. This is the case particularly for marginal social groups and lower social classes who cannot afford private health care. Despite Poland being seen as an economically very well developed country, there is the huge problem of the health care system and of education. These are not subsidized and the health care system actually tends toward catastrophe.

Other evident examples come from the transplant industry. In 1968 the Harvard Commission preparing a new definition of death clearly gave two reasons for the need for a new definition, 1) the burden of costs of keeping alive a person who is in coma or has irreversible brain damage; 2) ambivalent criteria of death could follow controversies around transplantation (Singer 1997, p. 34). Thanks to the new definition new possibilities for saving life through taking organs from dead patients appeared. The Harvard Commission admitted that the decision about the time of death was arbitrary, the moment when organs are still useful for transplantation was chosen (Singer 1997, p. 36). Biopower has good arguments for a continuation of biopolitical display by neoliberal ideas of quality of life: saving lives of organ recipients and concealing the differentiation between life worth living and life which is unworthy of being lived.

Yet the consequences of the transplantation business called forth an ethical critique. Dorothy Nelkin, in one of the first detailed analyses of this market, claimed that biotech companies reduce and decontextualize the body, deprive it of cultural meanings and personal relationships, reduce the body to a utility object (Andrews and Nelkin 2001, p. 5). Scott Carney warns Western societies of the absolute commodification of the body leading to the emergence of the "red market": the illegal sourcing and selling of organs. Today, the body can be treated as a set of exchangeable parts: organs (lungs, heart, kidneys, pancreas, intestines), tissues (cornea, skin, bones, bone marrow, ligaments), reproductive elements (sperm, embryos, placenta, embryos), as well as blood, plasma and hair. The corpse can be a luxury commodity worth more than 230 thousand dollars—writes Lesley A. Sharp (2006, p. 11). Only the richest can afford to undergo transplantation due to the cost of operations (Sharp 2006, p. 51). The growing demand for organs resulting from the improvement of surgical techniques, and the growing number of physicians specializing in transplantation attracted by high incomes and the creation of new transplant clinics, are compared to the symbolic form necrophagia and neocannibalism (Youngner 1996, p. 35). To avoid such associations, transplant professionals invented euphemistic language, which hides the process of commodification of the body (Sharp 2006, p. 12). This discourse is built around the rhetoric of exchange, a "gift of life," which is supposed to sublimate a strictly economical account. However, this narrative lacks a vital element that we know from Marcel Mauss' theory of exchange (1973): the principle of reciprocity. The lucrative transplantation industry resulting from the high value of organs and tissues is presented in terms of the cost of services (expenditure related to the acquisition of the body, transport, pre-and post-operative care, immune-suppression, hospital administration), yet discussion of the financial value of organs is taboo. Some economists and doctors believe that legalization of the body trade will solve the problem of "red market" crime and provide a greater supply of organs (Becker and Posner 2013, pp. 93–98). However, this utilitarian approach is criticized as leading to the commodification of the body to an absolute degree. One of the critics of bioeconomy is Michael Sandel, who writes that "we are heading towards a society where everything is for sale" (Sandel 2012, p. 21), which causes the loss of ethical values in relationships between people, and the expansion of inequality in relation to their level of health. According to Sandel, such goods as health, education, family life, nature, art, and civic duties should not be subject to the law of a market which destroys the very essence of the community. The human body is the last bastion to be conquered by the political economy of neoliberalism. All goods—living conditions, education, and art—have been seen as accumulated capital and have been captured in economic terms. Only the body and its parts as objects in the global market arouse hot disputes. On the one hand, we have the economic calculations of industry in terms of supply and demand and, on the other hand, the arguments of opponents of body economization.

During pandemic time moral questions appeared: if and how to protect the most vulnerable social groups? Nursing homes—not only in Poland, but also in Great Britain, Austria, Germany and other countries—became "death homes" due to a lack of proper end-of-life care. In Great Britain and Sweden the political strategy to avoid lock down, in consequence meant sacrifice of old people in favor of economy.

Social and economic inequalities

Commodification of "life itself" brought the body under the sway of neoliberalism where social inequalities are growing. The state withdraws from many areas of social supply and even those spheres which were at the beginning under control of the state began to be influenced by processes of privatization, e.g. education, art, environmental pollution and health.

Although in theory neoliberalism was supposed to reduce poverty and guarantee human rights for all, "individuals lack the financial resources to pursue their own rights" (Harvey 2007, p. 177). Sunder Rajan (2006) shows with the example of a clinic in India how "biocapitalism" reproduces traditional forms of exploitation of developing countries and is in fact neocolonialism. Developing countries and countries from the Third World, because of low costs of research and production, are good places for laboratories. Because of poverty it is easy to encourage people to take part in pharmaceutical tests. Such people become the "guinea pigs" of experiments but they do not benefit from these studies. The "invisible hand of the market" is producing new demands and new supplies. Styhre points out that "surrogacy is an alarming example of a gendered, neocolonial practice" (Styhre 2012, pp. 3207–3223). He refers to research in India which is "becoming a leader in providing surrogacy, and the term 'reproductive outsourcing' captures the very content of this trade" (Styhre 2012, pp. 3205–3221). Carney (2014, pp. 133–148) portrays how the surrogacy business changes the natural process of giving birth to a production process arranged in special closed centres where women are monitored and treated as incubators. He also reports how demand for children in aging populations is giving birth to a "red market" of oocytes and children designed for adoption. Didier Fassin (2006) shows up how "the right to make live" is transformed into the right to prolonged life for the upper class, allowing shorter lives for the working class who lack access to specialized services. But no government would admit that. Promoting further commodification of biology and scientific knowledge increases social inequalities and continues to concentrate the wealth of those who mainly benefit from biotechnology.

Aging populations and rising of treatment costs

Many authors have been sending warning signals, in an apocalyptic tone, about an unprecedented aging of the human population and the consequences of this process, which require political, economic and social responses (Andrews 2005, p. XVII). Europe is considered to be among the main regions where the aging of the population has reached an advanced stage. The aging of the population is accompanied by the so-called "double aging" of the European population, i.e. an increase in the percentage of the elderly is accompanied by an even faster growth in the number of people aged 80+, named the Fourth Age.

At the same time the capitalisation of health and life in the form of economic calculations has revealed the facts of excessive financial resources assigned to supporting life. John Saunders (1994, p. 78) notices that the most expensive ward is the ICU where cardiopulmonary resuscitation (CPR) absorbs much of expenditures and "the costs of maintaining a patient in the persistent vegetative state are enormous." The revolutionary results of biotechnology are praiseworthy but they are accessible only to the richest and are burden on public hospitals keeping people alive without the possibility of recovery.

All these processes take place in neoliberal conditions where since the 1980s, and subsequently, public sector activity such as health care has been weakened (Styhre 2012, p. 1316). In neoliberal ideology patients are regarded as consumers who themselves are responsible for their health. "Neoliberalism replaces an ethic of state care with an emphasis on individual responsibility and market fundamentalism […]. Health maintenance becomes a responsibility or a duty rather than a right" (Pitts-Taylor 2010, pp. 639–670).

A good example of the consequences of "medical neoliberalism" (Fischer 2009) or in other words "biomediated capitalism" (Pitts-Taylor 2010) is provided by Poland. In Poland, the population aging process is among the fastest and deepest in the EU because alongside the demographic processes that occur across the whole of Europe, Poland is affected by intensifying emigration coupled with a much lower intensity of immigration. Over the next few decades, Polish society may transition from being the youngest to the oldest in Europe (Okólski 2010, p. 69). Starting from the beginning of the 1990s Poland underwent political and economic transformation, and neoliberalism became an ideal model for governments and economic leaders. Medical care was included in the privatization process with outsourcing of medical services. Polish health care is a leader in the development of the private hospital sector. Measuring by the number of hospital beds, within 15 years private hospitals constituted one fourth of all hospitals (Sześciło 2017, p. 157). Private specialist health care is becoming the only accessible sector. For example, the average waiting time for a visit in a public cardiology clinic amounts to about 100 days, and in a public rehabilitation room—300 days. Generally the waiting times for visits to a public specialist and specialist tests are growing. This is because specialists migrate or move to the private sector where salaries are much higher. Even in private clinics there is also problem of dramatic shrinking of numbers of doctors and nurses as they age or migrate to Western countries. The consequence of neoliberal politics in health and social care and of population aging is the collapse of Polish end-of-life care. According to studies on formal and public care, the actual situation of the elderly and their families has been constantly deteriorating. Poland is among those EU countries where the satisfaction of care-related needs of dependent elderly people is at one of the lowest levels. Only one in twenty elderly people in need of care receives community care services (Tsolova and Mortensen 2006). In the Global Age Watch Index, Poland was classified in the 62nd place out of 91, and ranked last among European Union member states. Although the number of patients in LTC facilities has been growing since 2009, formal care remains underdeveloped in Poland. The increase in institutionalized LTC patients was observed only among stationary care patients, while home care provision has decreased. Residential stationary care is better developed, although with just 17 beds in LTC institutions per 1000 of the population aged 65 years old and over Poland has the lowest number of institutional beds per 1000 persons for LTC facilities in the entire OECD (2011). What we observe in Poland is reminiscent of non-voluntary euthanasia spread over time. Of course it is not euthanasia as the term means conscious agreement of the patient and a chosen moment of death, but the oldest and poorest are destined to extinction.

Conclusions

Doubt in the omnipotent knowledge of experts, pluralisation of social norms and bioethical views, blurring of the borders of crucial categories, such as aambiguity of the border between life and death, uuncertainty in life sciences and medical practices, *aporia* of economization of dying, "a heterogeneous multiplicity of the living" (Derrida 2008, p. 31), or more precisely abandonment of reframing life of human being as in opposition to other living species, but to assuming life as biodiversity of all species containing life and death are shaking the foundations of biopolitics.

Today, there is a struggle on the borders, on the thresholds that I mentioned above. Hybrids' vulnerability to being shifted, flexibility, and in fact the *uncertainty* about their place and definition, forms the main argument that there is a process undermining biopolitics. At least we can see that biopolitics is becoming problematised, from one side because of accusation of eugenics in the case of genetics, and from the other side because of the revelation of the limits of economy in the name of life necessity. We live in a culture on the edge, with a collapse of the traditional framework of life and death, and loss of the symbolic reference of institutions, whether they are churches or the modern state.

References

Agamben G. 2008a. *Homo sacer. Suwerenna władza i nagie życie* [Homo Sacer: Sovereign Power and "Bare Life"]. Warszawa: Prószyński i S-ka.

Agamben G. 2008b. *Co zostaje z Auschwitz* [Remnants of Auschwitz]. Warszawa: Sic!.

Andrews L., Nelkin D. 2001. *Body Bazaar: The Market for Human Tissue in the Biotechnology Age*. New York: Crown Publishers.

Andrews G. 2005. Foreword. In *The Cambridge Handbook of Age and Ageing*, ed. M. Johnson, XVII–XIX. Cambridge: Cambridge University Press.

Baudrillard J. 2001. *Simulacra and Simulation*. Ann Arbor: University of Michigan Press.

Baudrillard J. 2007. *Wymiana symboliczna i śmierć* [Symbolic Exchange and Death]. Warszawa: Sic!

Beck U. 2002. *Społeczeństwo ryzyka* [Risk Society]. Warszawa: Wydawnictwo Naukowe Scholar.

Becker G., Posner R. 2012. *Nieoczywistości. Ekonomiczna teoria wszystkiego* [Uncommon Sense]. Warszawa: Wolters Kluwer.

Carney S. 2014. *Czerwony rynek* [Red Market]. Wołowiec: Czarne.

Catts O., Zurr I. 2016. The biopolitics of life removed from context: Neolifism. In *Resisting Biopolitics*, eds. S. Wilmer, A. Žukauskaitė, 135–157. New York–London: Routledge.

Devisch I., Hoyweghen I. 2011. A new era of medical consumption: Medicalisation revisited. *APORIA* 3(3): 16–21.

Derrida J. 2008. *The Animal That Therefore I Am*. New York: Fordham University Press.

Esposito R. 2015. *Pojęcia polityczne. Wspólnota, immunizacja, biopolityka* [Political Notions. Community, Immunity, Biopolitics]. Warszawa: Universitas.

Evans M. 1994. Against the definition of brainstem death. In *Death Rites*, eds. R. Lee, D. Morgan, 1–10. London: Routledge.

Farrell K. 1998. *Post-traumatic Culture*. London: The Johns Hopkins University Press.

Fassin D. 2006. La biopolitique nest pas une politique de la vie. *Sociologie et Sociétés* 38(2): 32–47.

Foucault M. 2010. *Historia seksualności* [History of Sexuality]. Gdańsk: słowo/obraz terytoria.

Foucault M. 2013. Right of death and power over life. In *Biopolitics. A Reader*, eds. T. Durham, T. Campbell, A. Sitze, 41–60. London: Duke University Press.

Franklin S. 2003. Ethical biocapital: New strategies of cell culture. In *Remaking Life and Death. Toward an Anthropology of the Biosciences*, ed. S. Franklin, M. Lock, 97–128. Santa Fe: School of American Research Advanced Seminar Series.

Gaylin W. 1974. Harvesting the Dead. *Harpers*. Available at: https://harpers.org/archive/1974/09/harvesting-the-dead/. Accessed: 23.09.2020.

Girard R. 2018. *Apokalipsa tu i teraz* [Apocalypsis Here And Now]. Kraków: WAM.

Hallam E., Hockey J., Howarth G. 1999. *Beyond the Body*. London–New York: Routledge.

Harvey D. 2007. *A Brief History of Neoliberalism*. Oxford: Oxford University Press.

Helmreich S. 2008. Species as biocapital. *Science as Culture* 17(4): 463–478.

Hogle L. 2003. Life/time warranty: Rechargeable cells and extendable lives. In *Remaking Life and Death. Toward an Anthropology of the Biosciences*, eds. S. Franklin, M. Lock, 61–96. Santa Fe: School of American Research Advanced Seminar Series.

Kubiak A. 2020. *Assisted Death in the Age of Biopolitics and Bioeconomy*. Cambridge: Cambridge Scholars Publishing.

Lemke T. 2010. *Biopolityka* [Biopolitics]. Warszawa: Sic!.

Lock M. 2003. On making up the good-as-dead in a utilitarian world. In *Remaking Life and Death. Toward an Anthropology of the Biosciences*, eds. S. Franklin, M. Lock, 165–192. Santa Fe: School of American Research Advanced Seminar Series.

Mauss M. 1973. *Socjologia i antropologia* [Sociology and Anthropology]. Warszawa: Państwowe Wydawnictwo Naukowe.

Mbembe A. 2018. *Polityka wrogości. Nekropolityka* [Politics of Enmity. Necropolitics]. Kraków: Karakter.

OECD. 2011. Poland Long-Term Care. Available at: http://www.oecd.org/health/longtermcare. Accessed: 21.07.2019.

Okólski M. 2010. Wyzwania demograficzne Europy i Polski [Demographic challenges of Europe and Poland]. *Studia Socjologiczne* 4 (199): 37–78.

Pitts-Taylor V. 2010. The plastic brain: Neoliberalism and the neuronal self. *Health* 14(6): 635–652.

Rajan K. 2006. *Biocapital: The Constitution of Postgenomic Life*. Durham: Duke University Press.

Rose N. 2007. *The Politics of Life Itself. Biomedicine, Power, and Subjectivity in the Twenty-First Century*. Princeton, Oxford: Princeton University Press.
Sandel M. 2007. *The Case Against Perfection: Ethics in the Age of Genetic Engineering*. Cambrige: Harvard University Press.
Sandel M. 2012. *Czego nie można kupić za pieniądze. Moralne granice rynku* [What Can't Be Bought. Moral Limits of the Market). Warszawa: Kurhaus.
Saunders J. 1994. Medical Futility: CPR. In *Death Rites*, eds. R. Lee, D. Morgan, 72–90. London: Routledge.
Sharp L. 2006. *Strange Harvest. Organ Transplants, Denatured Bodies, and the Transformed Self*. Berkeley: University of California Press.
Singer P. 1997. *O życiu i śmierci. Upadek etyki tradycyjnej* [Rethinking Life and Death: The Collapse of Our Traditional Ethics]. Warszawa: PIW.
Spicker S. 1996. ICU Triangle: The ethics of scarcity, the ideal of impartiality and the inadvertent endorsement of evil. In *Death Rites*, eds. R. Lee, D. Morgan, 91–101. London: Routledge.
Stallybrass P., White, A. 1986. *The Politics and Poetics of Transgression*. London: Methuen.
Styhre A. 2012. *Organizations and the Bioeconomy. The Management and Commodification of the Sciences*. New York, London: Routledge.
Sześciło D. 2017. *Zmierzch decentralizacji?* [Twilight of Devolution?]. Warszawa: Wydawnictwo Naukowe Scholar.
Tsolova S., Mortensen J. 2006. *The Cross-Atlantic Exchange to Advance Long-Term Care, European Commission and ARRP Conference on Long-Term Care*. Available at: https://www.files.ethz.ch/isn/38579/SR%202006-09%20Cross%20Atlantic%20Exchange.pdf. Accessed: 30.01.2020.
Youngner S. 1996. Some must die. In *Organ Transplantation: Meanings and Realities*, eds. S. Youngner, R. Fox, L. O'Connell, 32–55. Madison: University of Wisconsin Press.

Maria Onyszkiewicz

A Phenomenological Approach to the Problem of Posthumous Harm*

Abstract

The discussion on posthumous harm is focused primarily on the subject problem—the question whether it is reasonable to postulate the possibility of posthumous harm despite the lack of a subject who could experience it. Pitcher-Feinberg's argument is paradigmatic for this approach. Both Pitcher (1984) and Feinberg (1993) bring the problem into question about the meaning of the term *posthumous harm* and seek the right reference for it. This reference is, in their view, a violation of the *interest* of the deceased, which also continues after his death. Daniel Sperling seems to be the follower of this approach. He says that human exists in two ways: as a person who has cognitive capacities and self-awareness and as a *Human Subject*, which holds interests (Sperling 2008).

I would like to expand these considerations and show, on the basis of phenomenology, that deceased in spite of their death continues functioning as an element of the structure of sense given to the world by those who knew them and, as such, may be the reference of the possible posthumous harm. For those close to them, they does not disappear but rather becomes *absent*, and that absence unlike non-being is something perceivable. In phenomenology the other is a fundamental condition of the intersubjective and objective world (Husserl 1960, 1989). The other and the ego together constitute a community which gives sense to that world and when the other dies the sense given to the world still needs him.

Keywords: posthumous harm, phenomenology, human subject, human body, death and dying

* The article is based on the author's MA thesis.

Introduction

A question of whether a deceased person can be harmed may seem absurd if a life after death is not assumed at first. As Epicurus pointed out: "that most frightful of evils, death, is nothing to us, seeing that when we exist death is not present, and when death is present we do not exist" (Epicurus 1987, p. 150). Many centuries later, a similar thought was expressed by Ludwig Wittgenstein—"at death the world does not alter, but comes to an end." He also claimed that "Death is not an event in life: we do not live to experience death" (Wittgenstein 2001, theses 6.431 and 6.4311, p. 87). In death we no longer exist, so our ability to learn and feel—including an experience of harm—cease to exist as well. However, the intuition that posthumous harm is plausible seems to be strongly rooted in our society—what is reflected for instance in a well-known maxim *mortuis nihil nisi bene.*

The discussion on posthumous harm took place mainly in the second half of the 20th century. It focused primarily on the problem of the subject—the question of whether the possibility of posthumous harm, despite the absence of a subject who could have experienced it, can be legitimately claimed. The aim of such an analysis of this issue was to explain the foundations of the intuition described above. It also tried to explore many reason for why it is so popularity shared.

The aim of this article is to discuss three possible approaches to posthumous harm: analytical, psychological and phenomenological. The first one, which has dominated the debate on posthumous harm, focuses on the subject problem. The second, shifts the focus from the deceased to his or her surroundings and loved ones. The third, which is my own contribution to the topic, makes use of the tools provided by Husserlian phenomenology and formulates a solution that to some extent reconciles the two previous ones.

The analytical approach

The representatives of the analytical approach prioritise the concept of the subject and ask the following questions: can the subject's problem be overcome? Is the subject necessary for the harm to occur? Is the concept of posthumous harm necessary, or should be rejected? I intend to discuss the analytical approach by analysing Pitcher-Feinberg's argument. I decided on it because it is the most frequently cited argument in the discussions. I also chose to mention Taylor's critique of this argument.

I call this approach analytical, because the solutions proposed in it are not about determining whether it is really possible to harm a deceased person, but about providing an appropriate reference to the concept of posthumous harm.

Pitcher's argumentation

George Pitcher based his argument on distinguishing between two possible descriptions of the deceased:

(a) description of an ante-mortem person (as a living person) after his death.

(b) description of a post-mortem person after his death (Pitcher 1984, pp. 183–184).

In the first description (a) we consider who the deceased was or what appened to they before he died at any stage of their life. In the second one (b), we refer to the deceased after their death—who they are, what happens to them when they are already dead.

Pitcher says that both, the deceased and the living person can be described in any way, but only the living person can be harmed. However, he states that a living person can also be harmed after their death, what can be expressed using the first type of description (a). To illustrate this thought, he gives the following example: "Mrs. Blue, now dead, was not in the least anti-Semitic, but that her spiteful neighbour now maliciously asserts that she was. This charge is a lie and since it is a lie about a person who is now dead, it may be said to constitute a wrong perpetrated against a dead person" (Pitcher 1984, p. 184). In Pitcher's opinion to lie about someone is to hurt the person about whom the lie is told, even if that person is dead. Mrs Blue is dead, but her neighbour harms her as an ante-mortem person. What the neighbour says is neither true nor false when referring to Mrs Blue as post-mortem person. False or true statements refer to Mrs Blue as a living (ante-mortem) person only (Pitcher 1984, p. 184). Pitcher points out that attributing the harm to Mrs Blue as an ante-mortem person on the basis of the events following her death seems to involve backward causation (Pitcher 1984, p. 185). However, he claims that this is only a guise. The event following a person's death does not involve the person's wrongs, but only makes the assessment of that wrongs true (Pitcher 1984, pp. 187–188). This means that if someone tells a lie about dead person, the lie does not cause a harm but just make it possible to attributed harm condition to that person (now dead). By analogy, he gives a hypothetical story of the President of the United States, Ronald Reagan: "If the world should be blasted to smithereens during the next presidency after Ronald Reagan's, this would make it true (be responsible for the fact) that even now, during Reagan's term, he is the penultimate president of the United States" (Pitcher 1984, p. 188). Pitchers claims that the end of the world make it possible to attribute to Reagan being the penultimate President of the United States. Being wronged, Pitcher says, can be attributed to Mrs Blue as an ante-mortem person the same way as being the penultimate President of the United States, to Ronald Reagan from the example. In this way, Pitcher is trying to overcome both the problem of backward causation and the problem of the subject.

Feinberg's argumentation

Joel Feinberg bases his argument on the concept of interest which he links with the notions of want, goal and aim. Preventing someone's wants, goals, or aims from being fulfilled is a thwarting of their owner's interest, which Feinberg identifies with harm (Feinberg 1993, pp. 176–178). He points out that the fulfilment or thwarting of a person's interest does not depend on their mental state—they do not have to face the fact that their want or goal has been thwarted, nor do they have to be aware of it (e.g. when someone does something secretly behind their back). As such, it can also take place after their death (Feinberg 1993, p. 181). Therefore, the concept of interest itself is sufficient to establish the existence of harm. This does not mean, however, that it is the interest itself that is the subject of the harm being claimed. It must always be able to be attributed to someone, to be someone else's interest.[1] In Feinberg's view, even if a person is dead, the interest can still be attributed to him or her—moreover, we do so even when we speak of a violation of the will of the dead (Feinberg 1993, p. 176). He follows Pitcher in this matter and assumes that the right person to harm is the ante-mortem. Acting against the will that was expressed in a lifetime, breaking promises and slandering the person after a death are considered by Feinberg to be against that person's interests and therefore to be harmful. To illustrate his position, he uses an example of "A women [who—M.O.] devotes thirty years of her life to furtherance of certain ideals and ambitions in the form of one vast undertaking" (Feinberg 1993, p. 181). He presents here three alternative scenarios:

> *Case A:* One month before she died, the "empire of her hopes" collapses utterly and she is personally disgraced. She never learns the unhappy truth, however, as her friends, eager to save her from disappointment, conceal or misrepresent the facts. *Case B:* The collapse of

[1] Feinberg himself points out here that his position has changed on this issue, because it was previously the interest that he considered as the right subject of harm (Feinberg 1993, p. 176).

> her undertaking and disgrace happen after her death. *Case C:* The undertaking collapses and the woman is disgraced during her lifetime. Before her death, a group of people made various promises to her about her undertaking. But when a woman dies, they break all those promises, tell lies about her and expose her secrets (Feinberg 1993, pp. 181–182).

Feinberg claims that it is intuitive and uncontroversial to acknowledge that harm was done to a woman in case A, even though the woman was unaware of it. He also claims that cases A and B are analogous, because in neither of them the subject is aware of the harm that was done to her. This means that there is harm in case B too (Feinberg 1993, p. 182). Feinberg points to Case C as peculiar, because a woman was not just harmed but she was wronged as well—she was betrayed and abused. And, in his opinion, harm is an important component of the wrong, so to wrong someone means to harm that person too (Feinberg 1993, pp. 182–183). Feinberg seems to consider it also uncontroversial and obvious.

Under the assumptions made by Feinberg the moment when the harmed condition begins becomes the key question—since what happens after a person's death does not cause this condition, but only makes the judgment of the condition true. According to Feinberg, that state begins when the first steps have been taken to fulfil a particular interest (Feinberg 1993, p. 186). That is to say, with the existence of an interest, the person automatically enters into a state of being harmed. If that interest appears to have been destroyed by future events—the occurrence of events that violate or completely destroy that interest is something that others find out about. As Feinberg puts it, the perspective of these people can be summarised by the following sentence: "From that point on (we now know) he was playing a losing game" (Feinberg 1993, p. 186).

Taylor's counterargumentation

James Stacey Taylor shows that the intuition behind the view that posthumous harm is possible can be clarified without involving this concept (Taylor 2005). First of all, it analyses Pitcher's attempt to solve the problem of backward causation. He notes that being the penultimate President of the United States is a sequential property (Taylor 2005, p. 314). The assertion about Reagan being the penultimate president is justified because he is element of a sequence (of successive presidents) to which this property relates. In his opinion, neither harm nor wrong are such properties. It is possible to harm or wrong a person if the action that causes it results in the loss of that person's well-being. It cannot be attributed on the basis of finding itself in a certain sequence. So there is no analogy between attributing to Regan the property of being the penultimate President of the United States and attributing to Mrs Blue the property of being harmed. That does not yet mean that it is impossible to find a good analogy. Pitcher himself assumes that it is possible to assign a living person certain property as a result of the events following his death.[2] However, he argues that the existence of such an analogy is insufficient to demonstrate that postulating the possibility of posthumous harm or wrong does not require backward causation. It still needs to be demonstrated that being harmed is a property of the same kind as that retroactively attributed (but without assuming backward causation) property (Taylor 2005, p. 315).

Next, Taylor analyses the Feinberg argument (Taylor 2005, pp. 316–317). In his opinion, the success of a woman's undertaking from cases A, B and C and her good reputation are not her only interests. It is also in her interest to be treated with respect and to preserve her autonomy as a person. In the case of A, woman's friends cheating on her about the collapse of her undertaking are thwarting her interests. By limiting her access to information to which she is entitled, they undermine her autonomy. While revealing the truth to her would probably not improve her well-being, hiding it has a clear impact on her life (which is ongoing) because she has been denied the opportunity to pursue her autonomy and the right to be respected by her friends. This impact explains why the harm can be attributed to her, even though she does not recognise it in her own experience. In cases B and C, the event described has no impact on a life of the woman (as she is dead) and therefore does not require postulating an occurrence of the posthumous harm.

Taylor also disputes with Feinberg's view that accepting that harm has been done entails accepting that wrong has also occurred. He presents the following example:

> If Bill offers to drive Ben to his early morning lecture and fails to show up, Bill wrongs Ben. However, if Ben's neighbour Betty drives him in instead, and if Ben were not inconvenienced or upset by this state of affairs, Bill did not harm Ben through wronging him. Since this is so, it is possible to agree with Feinberg that the dead can be wronged and deny that this shows that they can be harmed (Taylor 2005, p. 318).

Taylor try to explain the intuition behind attributing posthumous wrong to someone in a different way from the authors he discussed (Taylor 2005, p. 319). He points out that the statement "someone wrongs a dead person"

---

[2] Taylor describes the example proposed by Dorothy Grover: Mary and Joe shoot each other. They both shoot each other. However, Marry dies first, before the bullet she fires kills Joe. "Joe then dies after Mary. Joe's death thus makes it true that Mary was a killer, although this property could not be ascribed to her before her death." In this case, attributing property to being a killer, as a result of events following Mary's death, does not involve backward causation (Grover 1989, pp. 336–337; Taylor 2005, pp. 314–315).

can be understood as an expression of moral condemnation of the person who has done so. "For example, when John attempts to steal from David by putting his hand in his pocket. John engages in wrongdoing even if David's pocket is empty and John cannot steal from him" (Taylor 2005, p. 319).

Analytical approach—critique

These arguments, which are primarily engaged with the subject's problem, focus on linguistic considerations concerning the semantic framework of the concepts of harm (or wrong). After setting up that framework they ask about the possibility of applying these concepts to the deceased. They try to objectify harm. Objectifying harm is about indicating the conditions of the harm that does not involve the subject (in the sense that the subject does not have to be aware of it or experience it). Instead, they use the concept of interest. I want to underline that they do not face the question of whether a deceased person can be really harmed or whether posthumous harm exists in a metaphysical sense. They simply answer the question of whether a sentence stating that a deceased person has been harmed (after death) is a reasonable one. They examine whether a sentence have a logical value of truth or false—that is to say, they ask about the meaning of the phrase "posthumous harm."

With this approach with Ockham's razor, Taylor is right—there is no such thing as posthumous harm. However, this solution while rejecting the possibility of posthumous harm, does not solve all the problems associated with this issue. It leaves a question of the popularity of this intuition unexplained. Moreover, it does not provide any solutions for the problem of respecting the will of the dead.

On the other hand, one can agrees that the purpose of Pitcher and Feinberg's considerations was not so much to resolve the issue of the subject but only to clarify the basis of a fairly common intuition about the existence of posthumous harm. Then the solutions they proposed must be considered insufficient. Both of the scholars find answers to the question of the reference to the phrase "posthumous harm" interesting, but do not explain the reasons for its use. If the harm does not concern a person who has died (post-mortem), then why are some of us willing to talk about harming them? By saying so, do they really mean a certain interest or a person during her lifetime (ante-mortem)? Although the authors' proposals leave these and many other questions unanswered, the objectification they have made, the link between the concept of harm and the concept of interest, applies to the philosophy of law.

Posthumous harm in the philosophy of law

The problem of posthumous harm is considered in the philosophy of law in order to set the legal standards associated with the death of persons—such as respect for the will of the dead and posthumous copyright. Although the possibility of posthumous harm should perhaps be rejected in the metaphysical order, the existing legal order requires a more thorough examination of the issue.

Daniel Sperling, when considering the issue of posthumous harm in a legal context links the concept of harm to the concept of interest just like Feinberg: "An interest is a kind of stake in well-being of an object or state. It is the fact or relation of being concerned in something, which usually benefits or otherwise improves the prosperity of the interest-holder's state of affairs" (Sperling 2008, pp. 9–10). Then "harm is conceived as the thwarting, setting back, or defeating of an interest" (Sperling 2008, p. 10). He points out that, although the interest may survive the death of the person who was referred to, it must still be possible for it to be assigned to a subject during its lasting period. It cannot be a corpse (a post-mortem person), because as something inanimate, it cannot be an interest's holder. The ante-mortem person, on the other hand, no longer exists and as non-existent cannot have any interest either (Sperling 2008, p. 21). Since an interest is a part of the wellbeing of the subject, the harm must affect the subject by causing a change in it is wellbeing. The events described by Feinberg and Pitcher cannot change the wellbeing of the ante-mortem person, because the ante-mortem does not exist and what does not exist has no wellbeing and cannot be changed. We can think of the deceased as an ante-mortem person, but we cannot harm them. When we mention a deceased grandmother, we usually think of the person she was during her lifetime (as an ante-mortem person), not her remains (a post-mortem person), but our thinking does not change the person she was (Sperling 2008, p. 22).

Sperling also criticises the way in which Feinberg determines when the harmed condition begins. For the scholar it causes some contradictions. Even if we accept that Feinberg's solution does not involve backward causation, it is still not possible to identify the moment when the first action for the interest were taken in specific situations:

> What about the violation of one's reputation after death or the mutilation of one's corpse without notification of next-of-kin? [...] In other words, when do people invest in their good reputation or bodily integrity? Moreover, are people really expected to invest *actively* in such interests in order for them to be fulfilled or defeated? (Sperling 2008, p. 24)

The consequence of Feinberg's reasoning is to recognise that each of us is in a harmed condition because of our death—because it is in everyone's interest to stay alive (Feinberg 1993, p. 187; Sperling 2008, p. 24). This means that "the harmed condition exists well *before* the harmful event," what goes against common intuitions (Sperling 2008, p. 24). Sperling (referring to Callahan, whose concept will be presented in the next section; Callahan 1987, p. 345) notes the problem of responsibility for harm in the Feinberg concept: if it is possible to be harmed because of an event that has not yet occurred (which will happen in the future), it should also be possible to be responsible for it in the period preceding it (Callahan 1987, p. 345; Sperling 2008, p. 24).

Another consequence of Feinberg's proposal is that it is not possible to distinguish between the moment when someone is in a harm condition and the moment when he/she is not (he refers to the words of Will Waluchow 1986, p. 733). The wrongful questioning of someone's good reputation after the death of some person (T_H) is an event because of which that person was in harmed condition at some point in their life (T_L). However, what happens if after a certain time after the harm was done (T_R) that harm is repaired and the good reputation of the deceased is returned? According to Feinberg's argumentation, we should admit that because of this event (repair of the harm) the person was not in the state of being harmed at a point in their life (T_L). This means that the person at some point in life (T_L) at the same time was (due to a harmful event in T_H) and was not (due to a repairing event in T_R) in the harmed condition (Sperling 2008, p. 25; Waluchow 1986, p. 733). If we want to avoid such contradictions, significant changes should be made to the Feinberg concept, which would make it possible to clearly identify when a harmed condition begins and ends. It seems, however, that this would mean rejecting one of his basic assumptions, according to which harm is not an event but a process.

Sperling states that "there are different forms under which one can exist. I can exist materially as a physical being in the form of an 'aggregate of cells', and/or in a non-material way as a 'man', a 'person', a 'human being', etc." (Sperling 2008, p. 34). Some of them are merely imaginary constructions symbolising the moral or legal status of their holder. For example "the concept of a 'person' is a creation symbolising a subject who usually has cognitive capacities and self-awareness and is accorded with legal rights" (Sperling 2008, p. 35). In fact, he says, there is no such thing as a person—it is just a way of describing the subject. What really exists is a certain body with its own physical and mental states. When someone dies, we stop describing that body as a person because it loses the reason to attribute to it certain properties that we associate with being a person (e.g. self-awareness). Another way of human existing is, as Sperling proposes, existence as a *Human Sub-*

ject—„the subject *holding* all human interests *belonging* to the person whose interests they are" (Sperling 2008, p. 35). Even when she or he is already dead.

Sperling admits that interests related to a person may continue after their death (when they no longer exists), but also before their birth (when they does not yet exist). He therefore introduces four categories of interests depending on the period in which they occur (Sperling 2008, pp. 13–15): *pre-birth interests* that occur before birth, when person doesn't exist yet; *life interests* which span during personal life, from birth to death; *after-life interests* that stand after death, when a person no longer exist; *far-lifelong interest*—interests from second and third category. Because a person exists only during her lifetime and only then she can be a subject of interest, human subject is an interest holder before and after that time. Existing as a human subject is *persistent*—there is no moment to end it, but, like a person, it lasts in time and it is non-material (Sperling 2008, p. 36). A person is the owner of the interests because it is who, by reason of his or her mental and intellectual capacities, can be given legal rights. The human subject only holds them *on their behalf* when they no longer exists or does not exist yet. The human subject has no mental qualities but "its significance lies in the fact that this subject belongs to the moral community of humans." Furthermore its members "are bestowed with an entitlement merely to hold interests for the person whose interests they are, the defeat of which may constitute legal harm" (Sperling 2008, p. 37). A person, on the other hand, has a legal right to ensure that her interests are not unjustifiably thwarted—she is legally protected from being harmed—and the human subject who holds her interests is the logical construct for the realisation of that right (Sperling 2008, p. 38).

The psychological approach

Joan C. Callahan presents a different perspective from the analytical one (Callahan 1987). She takes a point of view that where interest described by Feinberg and Sperling continues despite the death of its owner in so far as it has been transferred to other (living) persons (Callahan 1987, p. 344). It no longer applies to the deceased, but to those who identify with them and consider their interest to be their own. Therefore, thwarting this interest is harmful to its living representatives, not to the deceased.

Callahan criticises Pitcher-Feinberg's argumentation based on the distinction between the description of the deceased as an ante-mortem and a post-mortem person. As it was said, the acceptance that an event occurring after the death of a person makes it possible to conclude that the person was harmed as an ante-mortem person (i.e. while still alive, before the harmful event occurred) is problematic. It leads, in its view, to the acceptance of an analogous reasoning for attributing responsibility for harm before harmful event (Callahan 1987, p. 345). This means that it would be possible to attribute responsibility to the person who caused the harm before taking the action resulting in the harm. It is a fatalistic vision that the harm actually does not depend on the offender or the person to whom it is done—what in Callahan's view, rather supports the idea that the dead cannot be harmed.

Callahan claims that an intuition about the possibility of harming the deceased is based on our psychological attitude towards them. The feelings we had for our loved ones when they were alive do not disappear after their death, so we are willing to continue to treat them as living (ante-mortem) persons (Callahan 1987, p. 347). This is an almost automatic empathetic reaction that enables us to identify ourselves with others, even after their death (Callahan 1987, p. 348).

She takes a psychological perspective on this issue because, in her view, there are no philosophical reasons for claiming that the deceased may be harmed (Callahan 1987, p. 348). Only from a psychological point of view one can identify oneself with the deceased as once alive, feel sorry for them and thus not be accused of being ridiculous. This does not require postulating the actual occurrence of posthumous harm.

Callahan suggests that her approach makes it possible to formulate arguments which, without addressing the issue of posthumous harm, justify the requirement to respect the will of the deceased and to keep the promises made to them before their death (Callahan 1987, pp. 350–351). In her opinion, the pre-mortem wishes of the dead are associated with a feeling of duty on the living when we attribute certain attitudes or recognise that they identify with certain values. We would not feel obliged to do so in her opinion in the case of a woman who wants to be buried with all her possessions. If, on the other hand, her wish were only to distribute her wealth to the living, Callahan claims this feeling of duty would probably occur (Callahan 1987, p. 350).

Although Callahan's argument is philosophically underdeveloped, her proposal is worth appreciating because of the new approach to the problem. She is redirecting attention from the deceased to the living—talking about posthumous harm does not, in her opinion, say anything about the deceased, but about the attitude of the living. However, Callahan does not discuss in an extensive way what that relationship is about. She stops at a psychological explanation, while from a philosophical point of view, it is interesting to ask about the basis of empathy that Callahan claims for the dead. In other words, Callahan's argument ends where philosophical argumentation should begin.

The phenomenological approach

In Husserl's phenomenology, the flesh [*Leib*] is the constitutive factor of knowing reality. It is a tool of will and a holder of sensations (opposed to the body [*Körper*] which is a material, physical object).[3] Ego acts through flesh and it is what sets its unique perspective on the world (Husserl 1989, pp. 151–154). At the initial level of the constitution, every experience belongs to ego's flesh and creates a sphere of its owness (Franck 2014, pp. 34, 79–80; Husserl 1960, pp. 95–96). As Didier Franck points out, within the sphere of owness, everything is here (in *absolute* here), there is nothing external for ego (Franck 2014, pp. 82–84). The perception of anything as external to the flesh, and perception of flesh as embedded in the external world as a body comes from the Other (Franck 2014, pp. 110, 112). Other, who is a flesh too, is something to which we do not only refer intentionally, but something that responds to our reference and also refers intentionally to us. In this way it sets the boundary for the sphere of ownness and gives the world a sense of something external, objective and mutual for ego and other (Franck 2014, p. 186). Ego recognises then it's flesh as a body embedded in the world just like other objects. In this way the ego is constituted as a psychophysical unity.

Intersubjectivity

As Husserl says, constitution of the other is the first step in a process of "a universal superaddition of sense to my primordial world, whereby the latter becomes the appearance 'of;' a determinate 'Objective' world, as the identical world for everyone, myself included" (Husserl 1960, p. 107). Then "as the transcendental 'We,' it [the transcendental intersubjectivity—M.O.] is a subjectivity [*Subjektivität*—M.O.] for this world and also for the world of men, which is the form in which it has made itself Objectively actual" (Husserl 1960, p. 107). The sense of the intersubjective world is therefore no longer created within the transcendent ego, but within the transcendent We, that is, together with the Other: "*Something that exists is in intentional communion with something else that exists.* It is an essentially *unique* connectedness, an actual community and precisely the one that makes transcendentally possible the being of a world, a world of men and things" (Husserl 1960, p. 129).

---

[3] German word *Leib* is translated in English philosophical literature in various ways. Most popular English equivalents of it are: "animated organism," "flesh" and "Body."

The first such community and is, according to Husserl, "The first thing constituted in the form of community, and the *foundation for all other intersubjectively common things*, is the *commonness of Nature*, along with that of the *Other's organism* and *his psychophysical Ego*, as paired with *my own psychophysical Ego*" (Husserl 1960, p. 120). While in the constitution of a common objective nature, the other appears as a transcendental condition of its possibilities, it must participate as present in the creation of the meaning of successive layers of the intersubjective world. Comparing this to the tactile constitution of one's own living body, Franck points out that the reference to the flesh of the other happens in the con-tact[4] i.e., a direct relationship with it (Franck 2014, p. 145). The other co-constituting world is therefore not something abstract, anonymous to ego, it is perceived as a concrete flesh with which ego interact directly. This relationship leads to the creation of a community of the ego and the other, their common world, to which a common sense they attribute. From that moment on, the sense of the world is closely connected with the other, even permeated with it. That sense is no longer a sense only for the ego, but is common, intersubjective. The community of the we transcends each of the subjects involved by producing a sense ascribed to the same world. Other, with whom ego relates are therefore the foundation of our perception of the world, metaphorically speaking, they are the prism through which we look at the world.

Death of the other

When the other dies, his body does not fulfil the sense of flesh, animated organism and subjectivity attributed to it. The con-tac is no longer possible because the intentional reference to it does not get a reflexive character, and the we—which he was a part of—lose one of its foundations. The world, which until now was common to the ego and the other, becomes a world only of the ego, which thus loses the possibility of transcending itself through a sense-creating we. However, the world as such, already constituted, does not disappear, but the sense given to it by the we becomes "empty." The world thus constituted in that way (with the other) demands the other, who co-created it. However, the other cannot appear because he is already permanently *absent*. His *absence* is not some kind of a non-existence which cannot be the object of perception or intentional reference. Instead it is precisely an *absence* "too discloses being" as Sartre wrote (Sartre 1978, p. xlix). Unlike non-being, it is something that can

[4] Jacek Migasiński, Polish translator, points out that there is a wording used by Franck: French words *tact* and *contact* mean "touch" and "contact" (Franck 2017, p. 187).

be seen. To illustrate this thought, he gives an example of a visit to a cafe where he met with his friend Peter. Being late a quarter, he notices that Peter is not in the café (Sartre 1978, p. 9). Sartre then perceives Peter's absence because he expected to meet him there. Without expectation, the *absence* cannot emerge (that is why he will not notice the absence of other people he did not expect to meet there). Although on a conscious level, we cannot expect to meet the deceased, we do expect this on the basis of our experience, habits and impulses. Our experience is a results of a sense given to the world in which constitution he participated as *present*. The common space appears to be associated with the deceased, although no longer finding the proper fulfilment of his possible or actual *presence*. Not all others can therefore be seen as *absent*, but only those who participated in the constitution of that part of the world relevant to the context. Floris Tomasini, referring to Sartre's concept, calls the absence of a dead loved one *existential absence*. Whereas the associated feeling of emptiness she calls *embodied loss* (Tomasini 2008, 2009). He says that "[e]xistential absence is an absence that obtrudes through our experience of the human condition and plays a central role in the understanding of phenomenology. There are different kinds of existential absences in relation to the human condition" (Tomasini 2008, p. 262). Another manifestation of existential absence which he analyses is parallel to the feeling of absence of a deceased person. He takes a case of a phantom limb syndrome, which can occur after amputation. Just as a person after surgery can feel his limb as existing but "shell like," "empty," despite being aware of its absence (Tomasini 2008, p. 251), a person after the death of someone close can feel his or her absence in similar terms as present somehow. A similar analogy is also proposed by Merleau-Ponty (1996):

> The man with one leg feels the missing limb in the same way as I feel keenly the existence of a friend who is, nevertheless, not before my eyes; he has not lost it because he continues to allow for it, just as Proust can recognize the death of his grandmother, yet without loosing her, as long as he can keep her on the horizon of his life. The phantom arm is not representation of the arm but the ambivalent presence of an arm (Merleau-Ponty 1996, p. 81).

This ambiguous presence is in his view a result of a commitment by the ego to the world as it was shaped for the ego—still taking into account the amputated limb or the deceased person who participated in his constitution. Although patients with phantom limb experience, as well as those facing the death of their loved ones, learn to function in a new situation and to some extent get used to their condition. Both the removed limb and the deceased remain in a person's "life horizon." The sense she has given to the world so far is closely linked to her body and flesh and to the people she met in it. To become familiar with the new situation requires that new senses be given to her world, but this does not necessarily mean that the earlier ones are cancelled.[5] The meanings associated with the deceased cannot be cancelled or forgotten, but should find a new place in the structure of meanings ascribed to the world. So as not to refer to the physical but symbolic presence of the deceased.

Posthumous harm in the phenomenological approach

The attachment to the others and feelings we have for them cause certain expectations about how these people should be treated. Since after death this attachment and those feelings do not fade away and may even intensify we can still have expectations about them (Tomasini 2008, p. 259, 2009, p. 446). According to Tomasini, posthumous harm is related to these expectations—thwarting them is, in the eyes of those who have them, harming the deceased (Tomasini 2008, pp. 259–260, 2009, pp. 447–448). In his opinion, a feeling that the deceased was hurt is analogous to the feeling of pain in a phantom limb. This position is close to that of Callahan. They both place the posthumous harm in the experience of the living and consider their feelings towards the deceased's loved ones as the basis for this. The difference is that Callahan seems to think that what is called posthumous harm is in fact harm done to living people who identify with the deceased and have feelings for the deceased—and therefore take over some of their interests. For Tomasini, posthumous harm refers to *absent* deceased persons and it is experienced as *existential loss*. However, there is still the problem of how someone who is not there can be harmed.

When the loved One dies, we lose the community of we. Then the sense that we have given to the world through it loses the fulfilment of his presence and becomes empty. However, the *emptiness* of the Other is not abstract but real even tangible and is experienced as an *embodied loss* because it refers to the impossible presence of the Other. This ambiguity of the experience of the Other's *absence* is the result of the involvement of the ego into the world as it was shaped for the ego. It still takes into account the deceased, who participated in its constitution, because the deceased remains in the "horizon of life" of the ego. The structure of meaning ascribed to the world still include the Other. The Other is an element of that structure. And that element of the

[5] Even if a person after limb amputation, if he or she learns to function in a new way and thus give new meanings to the world, he or she does not completely replace its earlier established together with others. After the loss of a leg, the stairs are still used to move between floors; after the loss of a hand, the keyboard is still adapted to writing on it with two hands, even though for a person after amputation it is an obstacle or impediment.

structure is the reference to the posthumous harm. Both the perceived absence of the deceased and his or her harm are not something that takes place objectively in the world—they only take place in the experience of people connected with the deceased, because the structure of meaning they attribute to the world includes him or her.

Conclusions

The aim of this article was to provide a phenomenological view of posthumous harm. Although a deceased persons cannot actually be harmed, they still functions within the structure of the sense of the community of which they was a member. As such is still perceived by their relatives as vulnerable to harm.

What has been shown here is how the death of significant others affects our perception of the world and, therefore, our functioning. The death of a loved one makes the structure of the sense attributed to the world no longer suit it—the senses associated with the deceased are no longer properly filled. The sense attributed to the world must be reconstructed so that the absence of the dead is not experienced as an embodied loss. This new image of the world is a reconstruction, not a complete novelty—it does not cancel the previous experiences, but changes their sense, situating them anew in the structure of sense attributed to the world. This reconstructed image of reality is not a finished work, but it is closely related to current events, which in certain circumstances may force a new correction of the image of the past, which in turn will affect our current perception of the world and our emotional attitude towards it.

References

Callahan J. 1987. On Harming the Dead. *Ethics* 97(2): 341–352.

Epicurus. 1987. Letter to Moenoeceus. In *The Hellenistic Philosophers*, eds. A.A. Long, D.N. Sedley. Cambridge: Cambridge University Press.

Feinberg J. 1993. Harm to others. In *The Metaphysics of Death*, ed. J.M. Fisher, 169–190. Stanford: Stanford University Press.

Franck D. 2014. *Flesh and Body. On The Phenomenology of Husserl*. Transl. J. Rivera, S. Davidson. Bloomsbury Publishing.

Franck D. 2017. *Dwa ciała. Wokół Fenomenologii Husserla*. Transl. J. Migasiński, A. Dwulit. Warszawa: Wydawnictwo Naukowe Scholar.

Grover D. 1989. Posthumous Harm. *The Philosophical Quarterly* 39(156): 334–353.

Husserl E. 1960. *Cartesian Meditations. An Introduction to Phenomenology*. Transl. D. Cairns. Dordrecht: Springer Science Business Media.

Husserl E. 1989. *Ideas Pertaining to a Pure Phenomenology and to Phenomenological Philosophy. Second Book*. Transl. R. Rojcewicz, A. Schuwer. Dordrecht–Boston–London: Kluwer Academic Publisher.

Merleau-Ponty M. 1996. *Phenomenology of Perception*. Transl. C. Smith. New Delhi: Motilal Banarsidass Publisher.

Pitcher G. 1984. The misfortunes of the dead. *American Philosophical Quarterly* 21(2): 183–188.

Redfern M. 2001. *The Royal Liverpool Children's Inquiry*. MR/CJK/071100. London: The Stationery Office.

Sartre J.-P. 1978. *Being and Nothingness: A Phenomenological Essay on Ontology*. Transl. H.E. Barnes. New York: Pocket Books.

Sartre J.-P. 2007. *Byt i nicość. Zarys ontologii fenomenologicznej*. Transl. J. Kiełbasa et al. Kraków: Wydawnictwo Zielona Sowa.

Sperling D. 2008. *Posthumous Intrests. Legal and Ethical Perspective*. Cambridge: Cambridge University Press.

Taylor J.S. 2005. The Myth of Posthumous Harm. *American Philosophical Quarterly* 42(4): 311–322.

Tomasini F. 2008. Embodying loss and the puzzle of existence. *Sociological Review* 56(S2): 249–263.

Tomasini F. 2009. Is post-mortem harm possible? Understanding death harm and grief. *Bioethics* 23(8): 441–449.

Waluchow W.J. 1986. Feinberg's theory of "preposthumous" harm. *Dialogue* 25(4): 727–734.

Wittgenstein L. 2001. *Tractatus Logico-Philosophicus*. Transl. D.F. Pears, B.F. McGuinness. London–New York: Routledge.

Cultural Studies on Death and Dying

Zygmunt Pucko, Joanna Przybek-Mita

Life in the Living Death of Frida Kahlo and its Reflection in the Painter's Work

Abstract

The concept of *inner death* has a long and interesting history. Various concepts of this notion have been presented in philosophy, literature and psychiatry. One of the most important views is this promoted by Bruno Bettelheim. It is known in the scientific discourse as the "life in living death." Many people have experienced this phenomena at some stage of their lives and, depending on the circumstances, this condition may last for a shorter or longer period of time. In some cases, the state of living death can build up and become repeatable; in others it passes quickly and finally fizzles out. Nonetheless, it always causes great desolation and destruction to our psyche. It is an extremely traumatic existential experience that cannot be fully understood or described by means of language. Frida Kahlo was one of the people who experienced this phenomenon throughout her life. It was annihilating the internal structures of her existence from the early years of her life up to its final stage. Frida's works, treated as an attempt to overcome this state of soul, became her existential reaction to the havoc caused by living in death. With this kind of transgression she tried to defend herself against the invasion of nihility. Her paintings often reveal the narration of internal decline, being at the same time a record of her fight against it. The reflections presented in the article are of innovative character, since the case of Kahlo has not yet been considered in the aspect of life in living death from the philosophical perspective, nor described by phenomenological or existential language.

Keywords: life in living death, nihility, transgression, painting, mask

Introduction

The current debate on the theme of thanatology is quite clearly made up of many different threads. The motif of death in life, however, has somewhat receded into the background or has disappeared completely as an object of intellectual exploration. At the same time, this phenomenon is quite important and it is worth remembering.

The various manifestations of death experienced in life, also known as internal death, overlap in some respects with another form of death understood as life in "living death." This is likewise difficult to express and has many appellations. One of its most dangerous variants was to some extent identified and described by Bruno Bettelheim (2004). Thanks to his many years of therapeutic work with emotionally disturbed children, the doctor observed that in their inner worlds his young patients subsisted in a state of living death. It was the only way in which his young patients could exist. However, the original sources of this hitherto unknown mode of human existence lie not in the person, but rather beyond. This state of death is shaped either by the interweaving of oppressive circumstances or by another human being. Regardless of the cause, each destroys its victim, chasing the victim into the wilderness and making it a wilderness of itself. It banishes it to "nowhere," drowns it in a timelessness and leaves what is no longer there in itself face to face with the abyss of nothingness (Bettelheim 2004). The victim perceives him or herself in terms of "something" rather than "someone" and calls themselves "supposedly a person."

Bettelheim used the metaphor of exile to evoke both the state of devastation in the foundations necessary to build relationships with others as well as the scale of damaged subjectivity. Bettelheim discovered successive layers of internal devastation in his patients and became increasingly certain that the quintessence of their experience lay beyond the conceptual range of possible expression. Based on this perspective, he suggested that the dark meanderings of experiencing a living death are better illuminated by art than by a case study. A work of art makes elusive human truths more audible, visible, and recognizable (Danek 2012). They are brought to the surface by literary texts, musical works, sculpture and painting. By means of pictures, for example, the artist communicates in a figurative language about what he experiences. It enables the artist to illustrate how they believe they are affected by others or by fate and how they deal with this fact.

Based on Bettelheim's theses, most of Frida Kahlo's canvases may be classified as *magna operas* of this type. Through drastic modes of expression, the artist revealed her own internal and external landscape of life in "living death" as well as the path to its transcendence. The means she employed to convey these ideas were metal rods, thorns, skeletons, bones, tears, human and animal hybrids. According to Hayden Herrera, Frida set out to achieve several important goals in this way.

First of all, she wanted to ensure that the viewer not only saw the suffering depicted in her artwork but could also taste and smell the desolation to which it led (Herrera 2003). Secondly, she portrayed her state of mind in terms of the injuries suffered by her body. In Frida's works, her body is seen naked, lacerated, torn, broken, bloody, and partially dead, just like her mind (Herrera 2003). Third, she strove to emerge from the chasm of non-being and appear in the consciousness of others as a fully-formed person of flesh and blood. By means of the above-mentioned motifs, she turned her body upside down on canvas and exposed her imagination as if filtered through an x-ray. She went to great lengths to reveal each and every single ordeal and every act of suffering down to the last detail (Herrera 2003). Many researchers of Frida Kahlo's work believe that her paintings represent an intimate journal on the extreme tragedy of existence (Kulpińska 2016).

This landscape of a life in living death was already outlined at the very beginning of Frida's ontogenesis, when she first felt emotionally abandoned by her mother with whom she yearned to establish a bond (Grimberg 1993). Frida recalled that her mother never fed her as an infant, but instead employed a wet nurse exclusively to perform this task. There are many indications that the wet nurse treated breastfeeding as a source of income without being personally engaged with the baby. As is common knowledge, an infant can gauge early on the various emotions of its carers. When it is already six months old it begins to be aware of the interpersonal relationships taking place in its presence. The nature of those interactions significantly affects the emotional make-up of the child and either satisfies their needs or deprives them of them. In both cases, an emotional matrix is imprinted on their minds that has long-lasting consequences (Ericson 1959). We can posit the hypothesis that the aura of barrenness that Frida experienced at the dawn of her existence left its traces in her mental outlook in subsequent stages of her life, functioning as a Platonic anamnesis reminding of her underlying feeling of exile in an emotional wilderness. This impression undeniably had an impact on her, as she visualized it thirty years later in the painting "My nanny and me." The artist considered it to be one of her most expressive works (Kettenmann 2002).

A huge rupture in Frida's existence occurred at the age of six when she fell ill with polio, which confined her to bed for almost a year with limited social contact. Polio not only left Frida with a deformed foot and calf on her right leg. Her handicapped limb was also used as a pretext by Frida's peers to exclude her from their social circles (Cercená 2009). Frida was especially wounded by the spiteful nicknames they gave her. According to her biographers, henceforth Frida had a two-fold awareness of herself as an incomplete being. She realized that a crippled girl could not be like other children (Le Clézio 2010). At the same time, she also felt the drastic withering away of her own "I." Her inability to find a home in the cemetery of her own normative self-image and her feeling of loneliness compelled her to seek refuge in the world of imagination. There she created a perfect copy of herself without any flaws or defects. This concocted phantasy image became more real than the real Frida. It rose to the rank of a faithful confidant, mentor, permanent friend and sister.

The pages of her diary reveal a great deal about the role this fantasized double performed in Frida's dying psyche. They confirm the thesis that the artist never said goodbye to her phantom. What is more, this dream, shaped by this sense of thanatic wasting away, transformed into a second Frida (Le Clézio 2010), which compensated for all her deficiencies (Kohut 1977). Later in her life the artist gave her *alter ago* material form on a canvas bearing the title "Two Fridas."

A next event that doomed Frida to a living grave was the tragic trolleybus accident she suffered during her teens. We should add here this grave was not a real grave. Rather, as a result of this traumatic event, she became in a way her own tomb (Le Clézio 2010). Based on medical documentation it is know that her body was completely devastated (Le Clézio 2010). Surgeons spent hours putting back together her butchered body piece by piece. When they reset her bones, the immobilized Frida was laid flat on her back in a plaster corset surrounded by cardboard material. The box looked like a sarcophagus (Herrera 2003). The body encased in it turned into a microcosm of pain. Every breath was torture. Remaining motionless became an unbearable torment. Here was the terror of being utterly incapacitated, the despair at having no control over one's own body. This was the hell of loneliness, a hell that came from the constant recollection of those terrible scenes from the collusion. She was haunted by a fear of death accompanied by visual hallucinations. At night Frida would see the silhouette of death circling around her bed (Herrera 2003). She was oppressed by a sense of time standing still and every minute turning into eternal despair. It was a catastrophe in which all reference points were lost.

This coincidence of different episodes of extreme suffering led to the disintegration of the scaffolding that constitutes a person's individuality (Fimbel Di Giovanni and Lee 2019). Cast adrift and lost in herself, Frida suffered a total breakdown. When she woke up from this mental cataclysm, she knew that there would be no cure for her solitude anymore, and she knew the entire truth about her death. A careful reading of the artist's correspondence leads to the conclusion that from her perspective the deceased Frida was less dead than the actual Frida. In a letter to a friend from October 13, 1925,

Frida writes that *she will be a wreck for the rest of her life* (Herrera 2003).[1] The unfolding element of disintegration within herself had transformed her into a corpse-person which, although physically filling the space occupied by herself, was still more in death than in life. The state of being of this individual, eviscerated of the content of the personal "I," was akin to dying in the wilderness *of a painful planet, as transparent as ice* (Herrera 2003, p. 72). Frida found this experience of internal annihilation impossible to translate into visual form and thus never transferred it to the canvas.

The landscape of the artist's life in living death acquired a further sombre hue through a series of miscarriages. Because of the injuries to her pelvis and spine, Frida was unable to carry any pregnancy to term. Abortion always triggered a powerful somatic shock and bouts of proliferating despair. These were critical moments in which Frida experienced the height of suffering in its cruellest form, and in her mourning she reached the edge of an existential abyss beyond which she wanted to take the next step. She renounced life altogether and desired death.

Several of Frida's works highlight the extreme variations that life assumed at this stage of her living death. However, it is difficult to discuss each of them separately in this analysis. Nor is it necessary, given that the feelings and thoughts that Frida invested in these canvases revolved around one and the same theme. The two pictures that lie closest to this matrix of interweaved reflections are the lithography "Frida and the Miscarriage" and "Henry Ford Hospital," which make a shocking impression (Drucker 1991, p. 68).

Of all the seeds that contributed to the painter's state of living death probably the worst was Diego's affair with her younger sister Cristina and the annulment of the marriage. Her loss of Diego undoubtedly fostered an increasingly acute feeling of despair, which Paul Tillich called *despair within despair* (Tillich 1983, p. 58). Frida was aware that she was ebbing away in circumstances in which the best qualities of her soul were dwindling with her. The self shatters into small pieces, skills wane, talent dries up. Frida did not perceive this invasion of non-being in terms of her insignificance, condemning her to lead a half-life or to the loss of only part of herself, as some experts on the subject proclaim (Kettenmann 2002, p. 52). Rather, divorce reached down to the very foundations of her being and infected every fragment of it with the poison of counter-existence. The artist captured this genre of decay in "Two Fridas." Meanwhile, her self-portrait entitled "The Broken Column" served as an iconic panorama borne out of Frida's persistent stripping down of her existence in the declining phase of her life. The painting exudes terror and an unbearable tension. The spectacle of ruthless torment seems to burst

---

[1] An extensive selection of local correspondence follows the biographies of the pen in H. Herrera, *Frida. Life and Work of Frida Kahlo*. It is also the source of quotations quoted in the text.

through the frame of the canvas. The dissection of the body into two poles with jagged edges resembles the fissure formed after an earthquake.

As a visual narrative of the annihilation of a life in living death the "Broken Column" constitutes a special composition of signs and symbols. Its uniqueness is evident in the arrangement of these signs and symbols, which refer to objects, events and phenomena that are not directly present in the field of perception, but which are loaded with enormously powerful content in terms of both philosophy and martyrdom. The sharp, strong nails driven deep into the naked, subtle body are a symbol of suffering embedded in the situation to which it refers. Their topographic distribution is a reference to the martyrdom of St. Sebastian pierced with arrows (Kettenmann, 2002, p. 67). An even more powerful symbol of passion is the fabric wrapped around Frida's hips. Through this motif, borrowed from Christian iconography, the artist redirects our thoughts to the mystery of the suffering of Christ who, in his agony, was left with only the cloth around his loins (Kettenmann, 2002, p. 67). The loincloth of the Passion constitutes a *sui generis* epiphany of Frida's torment, a drama that is much more complex than one might think and at the same time remains impenetrable to the intellect.

Tears are an important component in the painting's architecture of signs and symbols. These inseparable attributes of Frida's existence, shed by mournful eyes down still cheeks, appear to articulate her despondency. In the scene before the viewer, besides suffering her tears suggest a "hint" of the weeping Madonna. The intriguing content of an anthropology focused on a life in living death, one of the main components of which is a sense of utter loneliness and hopelessness, is evoked here in the symbolism of the landscape. It merges with the inner landscape and constitutes its external environment. Both these dimensions are linked with and interpenetrate one other in a coherent stream. One appears to dissolve into the other and lose its substance as a separate entity. A dehumanized existence is lived out on a distorted earth and vice versa. Nature, hostile to life, impacts on existence and ravages it in its own image. The rocky crust, scorched by the sun, is a terrain without a continuous structure. We can see many dents, gaps, cliffs, chasms, pits, ravines, all identical to the open wounds in Frida's body. On the fringes of this ruptured universe looms *mulier dolorum* the light blue line of the sea. It is a sign of hope that reflects other headlands of existence and the possible fulfilment of various ideas about oneself. Unfortunately, the sea is too far away, It is beyond the reach of Frida, an artist tormented by a living death.

The logic driving the chronic, almost constant repetition of a life completed in a state of living death did not provide for an end point when Frida Kahlo's torment would cease. The repetition of disaster that descended upon the artist like an avalanche crushed her existence to a pulp until the very end of her time in this world. The last decade of her life was a truly apocalyptic period in particular. At the end of the 1940s Frida was forced to undergo another series of surgeries on her spine. She had to endure over thirty procedures throughout her entire life. She also suffered gangrene in her right leg as well as an infection that affected her entire body. Her right toes were eventually amputated. For weeks on end she was confined to a hospital bed, imprisoned in various corsets.

These moments felt like a clasp binding tightly the incomplete circle of a life of excess experienced as living death. Frida's response to this relentlessly oppressive way of being was to seek relief in painkillers, alcohol and drug addiction. After exhausting all coping outlets, she attempted suicide (Le Clézio 2010, p. 50). A few days before her death, Frida painted a picture on the last page of her diary, which she entitled "Time." The image depicted is one of almost apocalyptic chaos. The open sky, glowing with an intense pink light, is bathed in heavy rain that falls like teardrops. On the right side of the picture and moving towards the edge is a black angel wearing a gore-splattered, bloody crown and which is trying to flee this scene. Many experts believe that this is a visualization of Frida's self as she departs this world, while others see the angel as a personification of death. And yet what Frida was actually trying to say in this way, no one has yet been able to exactly determine. However, the words written next to the outline of the black angel and summing up her fate, leave no room for doubt: "I hope you are happy to leave, and I hope never to come back" (Le Clézio, 2010, p. 215).

Conclusions

The pessimism reflected in the paintings discussed above borders on the fatalism of an ancient tragedy. It would be risky, however, to persist with the idea that the theme of catastrophism present in the artist's canvases was nothing but a faithful reflection of the conditions of her existence. For Frida painting also had a redeeming value. It provided her with a key to understanding herself. It is difficult to argue with the view that Kahlo's works functioned as a bridge between emotional engagement in the world and a form of coexistence with other people. If we pursue this psychologically-slanted line of reasoning we discover more and more nuances to Frida's genius and its rather tangled coupling with her diminishing experiences (Lindauer 1999, pp. 2–9). This insight, although cognitively valuable, is not on its own sufficient to tackle the mystery underlying the transgression of life in living death.

Its singularities are perhaps better grasped by adopting a phenomenological approach. In the context of the events of her life, Kahlo's artistic work appears to be a struggle for existence (Herrera 2003, p. 71), a private war between "dead" Frida and living Frida wishing to live in her own right. Hence, many of Frida's works seem to be almost acts of being born anew and to a large extent constitute a space of self-creation. The visual and surreal manifestations of herself are a variation on a myth that was the opposite of who Frida really was (Zamora 1990, pp. 7–20). By means of these fantastical images, she became someone whom she wanted to be both in her own eyes and in the perception of others (Schaefer 1992, p. 7). For the most part she concealed the drama of this inner antagonism under a mask of peace and the majesty of human dignity rooted in the canon of the heroic *arete*. By means of the intentionality of the mask, Frida brought to the surface certain values and created features that she particularly desired to demonstrate, while at the same time highlighting the context in which they took shape. And with this mask, draped theatrically and combined with stoic apathy, Kahlo built up the steadfast figure of the Grande Dame of suffering, with which she identified so much that the mask began to reflect the profile of her own face and came to express a certain truth related to a specific situation (Fimbel Di Giovanni and Lee 2019). For this reason, in the artist's paintings, understood as an illustration of the artistic transgression of life in living death, real faces changed places with her masks and often merged into one (Thomson 2010, p. 218).

This translocation of masks and faces, and sometimes their mutual coherence, is the hallmark of Frida Kahlo's transcendence. By her commitment to transcending the conditioned, Frida Kahlo achieved a certain margin of independence. Through the act of transcendence, she captured on canvas the epic of a traumatic life in a state of living death and created her own masterpiece that has no counterpart in the art of painting.

References

Bettelheim B. 2004. *Uciekinierzy z życia. Leczenie dzieci zaburzonych emocjonalnie.* Warszawa: Wydawnictwo Akademickie Żak.

Cercená V. 2009. *Frida Kahlo.* Kraków: Wydawnictwo Zielona Sowa.

Danek D. 2012. *Śmierć wewnętrzna.* Gdańsk: słowo/obraz terytoria.

Drucker M. 1991. *Frida Kahlo. Torment and Triumph in her Life and Art.* New York: Bantam.

Ericson E. 1959. Identity of the life cycle. In *Psychological Issues*, ed. G.S. Klein. New York: International Universities Press.

Fimbel Di Giovanni J., Lee R.R. 2019. The art. And Suffering of Fida Kahlo (1907–1954). Available at: http://www.eapsp.org.au/files/the_art_and_suffering_of_frieda_kahlo.pdf. Accessed: 10.09.2020.

Grimberg S. 1993. Thinking of death. *Women's Art Journal* 14: 44–49.

Herrera H. 2003. *Frida. Życie i twórczość Fridy Kahlo.* Warszawa: Świat Książki.

Kettenmann A. 2002. *Frida Kahlo 1907–1954. Cierpienie i pasja*. Köln–Warszawa: Taschen/TMC Art.
Kohut H. 1977. *The Restoration of Self*. New York: International University Press.
Kulpińska K. 2016. Autoportret artystki w polskiej grafice na tle wizerunków własnych graficzek polskich i amerykańskich z lat dwudziestych–trzydziestych XX wieku. *AUNC Zabytkoznawstwo i Konserwatorstwo* 47.
Le Clézio J.M.G. 2010. *Diego i Frida*. Warszawa: Wydawnictwo Naukowe PWN.
Lindauer M.A. 1999. *Devouring Frida. The Art History and Popular Celebrity of Frida Kahlo*. Middeltown: Wesleyan University Press.
Schaefer C. 1992. *Textured Lives: Women, Art, and Representation in Modern Mexico*. Tucson: University of Arizona Press.
Thomson Z.B. 2010. The wound and the mask. Rape, recovery and poetry in Pascale Petit's The Wounded Deer: Fourteen poems after Frida Kahlo. In *Feminism, Literature and Rape Narratives*, ed. S. Gunne. New York: Routledge.
Tillich P. 1983. *Męstwo bycia*. Paris: Rebis.
Zamora M. 1990. *Frida Kahlo: Brusch of Anguish*. San Francisco: Chronicle Books.

Łucja Lange

Cancertainment. How Entertainment May Help People with (and without) Cancer?

Abstract

The main goal is to shed more light on the notion of "cancertainment" as a means of diffusing knowledge and reducing tension between those who suffer as a result of cancer and those who have only an exaggerated idea of the disease. I would like to focus on two questions: is cancer really entertaining (and if yes, for whom)? And how should cancer patients react to this name and its connotations?

I will try to present this issue from a broad perspective, discussing both the positive and negative sides of such "manipulation." How are cancer patients depicted in TV series? How do cancer patients see themselves? Can we learn anything from the portrayal of cancer in pop culture? And, most importantly, does cancertainment make any difference? Does it destigmatize cancer?

Keywords: cancer, suffering, patients, TV series, pop culture

Introduction

Any introduction to the subject of cancer and its cultural meaning requires highlighting a number of medical and sociological facts. The World Health Organization (WHO) states that "Cancer is a large group of diseases that can start in almost any organ or tissue of the body when abnormal cells grow uncontrollably, go beyond their usual boundaries to invade adjoining parts of the body and/or spread to other organs." This definition mentions any cause of cancer, as there are many and it is not clear if they lead to cancer in every case. Cancer remains a serious social problem, mainly due to the social losses that result from it. We can also read on the WHO website that "Cancer is the second leading cause of death globally, accounting for an estimated 9.6 million deaths, or one in six deaths, in 2018" (WHO 2021). The probability of getting cancer is high and will increase with the aging of society as a result of genetic and family conditions, an unhealthy lifestyle, and environmental threats.

A look at the data collected by the International Agency for Research on Cancer (IARC) two years ago shows that cancer is omnipresent throughout the world, although the data does not provide us with conclusive information as to the causes of cancer, what constitutes proper treatment and whether a person will ever be cured (Global Cancer Observatory (GCO)) (IARC 2018).

The WHO website also reveals a correlation between survival rates and such factors as the quality of available health care and early detection (WHO 2021). However, despite the fact that richer countries with better health systems appear better prepared for cancer, blogs written by their citizens reveal cases of patients being denied access to appropriate care due to being too young, or because they lack sufficient financial resources or support from others to undergo medical treatment. There were also cases of misdiagnosis and medical malpractice, and diagnoses that took so long that patients experienced unbearable stress waiting for the final results and "verdict." As a consequence, cancer issues are not unequivocal.

These issues also appear in many testimonies written by cancer patients and cancer survivors. They emphasize the fact that we know nothing or not much about the causes of cancer nor about the ways to cure it and the odds of cancer returning. One author and blogger who fought breast cancer, Mary Valle (2010), wrote:

> I've met plenty of young cancer patients who have "done nothing" to invite their cells to start mutating. Can we just admit it? We're in the midst of an epidemic and no one really knows what's happening, but I suspect it has something to do with environmental toxins, which probably can never be proven. Can we all just stop pretending that cancer is something unusual? And something that can be cured? A lot of people want me to tell them that I'm fine. That I'm cured. "You're fine, right?" they say, showing the worry lines on their faces, trying to feed me words I won't say. Because they want to know that they're going to be OK when they get cancer. Because they don't want to hear me say, "Nobody really knows what's going to happen once your cells start mutating."

She raises a number of important issues, such as the uncertainty, fragility and fortuity of cancer occurrence and the fear it engenders. That is why there is a need to tame it and make it "easier" for those who have cancer and those whose family members or friends are suffering from it. In addition to the subject of cancer as a terminal illness and a threat, nowadays, along with the increasing chances of successful cancer treatment, we are also dealing with something that we might call "a society of remission" "because more and more people live after being cured of cancer, and their experience of the illness and treatment is life changing and also needs to be addressed in sociological researches, culture and medicine" (Scambler and Scambler 2010).

This change in life prospects has occurred in tandem with changes in social roles. As a consequence, they may also result in a loss of social identity, which means that a person who does not know who she/he is in a social sense, does not know how to behave in certain situations. Tensions arising from a disturbance in a patient's social identity may also lead to their psychological and social isolation. Hence, one way of preventing such negative consequences is to ensure the patient has support—for example from family or friends. In addition, the disruption in a patient's living situation and behavior as a result of serious illness may cause the patient to find themselves excluded from their usual activities, thereby narrowing the scope of their social relationships. This is also the reason why cancer patients need information—they are trying to adapt to a new situation for which they are unprepared.

Cultural means of taming cancer can help address this need for information. Books, films, art, etc. can help people understand their situation and find their own way of dealing with it. But should all such sources be only informational in nature or can they be also entertaining? I will try to answer this question in the following paragraphs.

Is cancer hilarious?

Can an illness, any illness, be something we can joke about? There are people who find it helpful to laugh—no matter how hard it is and how unfavorable the results of treatment. All the absurdity of being a cancer patient (a victim of a disease) deserve a good giggle. It works not only for those who experience the pain and a state of constantly living with the unknown, but also for their families and friends. Cancer can be overwhelming and making jokes about it is somehow a cleansing experience.

Mary Valle is one of those who is critical of the idea of making cancer or rather making "the cancer fight" a topic for TV series and films. She says: "Cancer is bad enough without feeling exploited on top of it" (Valle 2010). Her article in *Killing the Buddha*, an online magazine of religion, culture, and politics, is a reaction to a TV show entitled "The Big C" and some of the scenes used to promote it in different magazines. She feels embarrassed and angry at the sight of Laura Linney playing the role of a cancer patient in the show, a sexy blonde who does not look like someone suffering from an oncological disease. She may be justified in her view as the main character in the series decides not to fight her illness, but instead mostly struggles with herself and the pressures of being a mother, wife, teacher, and cancer patient. She is trying to find herself in a new scenario—hence, she adopts the image of a gorgeous, attractive woman, as she resolves to live life to her full potential. Viewers who know the series will understand the pictures and images used to promote it. The character played by Linney decides to undergo treatment and her appearance changes. I understand Valle's point—the over aestheticization of cancer to sell the story on television is neither fair nor honest. But where in the entertainment business is there honesty and fairness? I am not even sure if it is possible.

On the other hand, we have many examples of young cancer patients like Heidi Schultz Adams (2008), who founded and created a safe space on the web to share stories, seek understanding, find answers and laugh together as sometimes there is nothing else one can do. Planet Cancer is the place where the word "cancertainment" first originated. There are lists of different kinds of popular culture creations on the theme of cancer and these are placed in a section called "cancertainment" (Planet Cancer). There are several books—the first and best known medium for sharing experiences of illness—movies and shows, music, comics, video games and so on. I could also add to this list blogs and art as they also perform the same role. The founders of a number of other websites decided to create their own content and "top ten" lists of songs, films and TV series, including stand-up comedy performances and books. Heidi argues that humor, such as the kind conveyed in cartoons depicting certain aspects of treatment, help patients and their families cope with illness as such cartoons break down intimidating experiences into "smaller, manageable, bite-size moments" (Szabo 2006).

In Poland we are familiar with the example of Katarzyna Kozyra (1996) and her "Olympia." Hence, the subject of cancer or illness in art is already well known, although mostly it is treated as a part of the healing process or a way of dealing with a specific condition. Art Museums in Lodz, Poznan and Warsaw have organized exhibitions on the subject of illness and cancer. In Poznan the exhibition was entitled: "Illness as a Source of Art." The curator's guiding principle was the assumption that an artist's illness is significant for their art, penetrates matter and reveals itself in various ways. Numerous works have been created in conditions of suffering, not as a way of coping with pain but rather as its manifestation. The experiencing of an artist's pain and suffering becomes in this case a kind of entertainment—"art reveals itself as one of the expressions of suffering, and not as a cure for disease" (Jowsa 2019).

However, art's influence on people is narrow and limited, while popular culture is more accessible. This fact is reinforced by the existence of "cancer celebrities" who fight for the cause and help popularize the subject. One such example is the actress Fran Drescher, who starred in the comedy series "Nanny Franny" ("The Nanny") and who was herself diagnosed with cancer. First, she was misdiagnosed and mistreated for other conditions, which led her to found her own organization called *Cancer Schmancer* which treats cancer as something to laugh at and promotes issues connected with healthcare and the early detection of cancer. Fran Drescher champions positive attitudes and maintaining a sense of humour (the Cancer Schmancer Movement).

Iva Skoch and Kairol Rosenthal (2009) are also advocates of a laughter-filled approach to the disease, they embrace the concept of "cancertainment" and suggest that young adults undergoing cancer treatment take a different approach to the disease than older generations. Liz Szabo (2006) states: "While some say there's nothing funny about cancer, a growing number of survivors and their families are using comedy to tell their stories."

To return to the question: is cancer hilarious? The answer is, no it is not. However, it can be treated with humor, simply as a way of dealing with the emotions and suffering that come with the illness. That is why cancertainment in its many guises remains popular and people resort to such ways of expressing themselves and learning more about cancer.

What is cancertainment?

The concept of cancertainemt was devised by young adults in their 1920s and 1930s, and is widely criticized by older cancer patients who like Mary Valle who feel shame and anger at the sight of yet another film or series about cancer starring aesthetically appealing actors, and who feel "raped" and "violated" by the experience of having the port put in or other kinds of treatment they undergo. Cancertainment was created around 1995 by Planet Cancer and meant "comedy about cancer treatment" (Planet Cancer). According to the definition provided by Planet Cancer cancertainment mostly consists of creations—pop culture creations such as books, movies, music, humor, video games, comic books and stand up comedy, tv series and blogs which offer inspiration, comfort and amusement to people (Planet Cancer).

It is also defined in the *Urban Dictionary* website as everything related to cancer in the broad sense of the term—the treatment, the drugs, the feeling that your own body has betrayed you, the politics, the bureaucracy, and the payments but also conversations about cancer and those notoriously vexing questions that do not help patients but rather mostly annoy them, such as "are you OK?" (FeakCitySF 2008).

There are many cancertainment creations worth mentioning—such as, for example, numerous comic books. Matthew Paul Mewhorter created "Cancer Owl" a very honest and sometimes rather oddly illustrated story in which he drew himself as an owl and explained "what it was like to have cancer" (Mewhorter). He wrote that:

> With cancer, there's no easy way to talk about it, so you might as well go all the way. Be you in all your glorious "you-ness" and to hell with those who don't have the stomach for it. Your pain matters! Your story matters! And all the sufferers of this damned disease who feel shamed into silence will see YOUR story and say, "Thank you!" and quite possibly get the courage to share their story and make a difference with someone else. So when you go to share your story, in whatever way you choose to share it, you might get an uneasy feeling about "what they might say." You might get downright terrified! These are normal feelings. But I think you'll be happier for taking the leap, speaking your truth, and making a difference (Mewhorter 2015).

Another noteworthy example is Miriam Engelberg's *Cancer Made Me a Shallower Person: A Memoir in Comics* (2006), which reflects the author's personal struggles and the truth about breast cancer according to Engelberg's own experiences. This is not simply another inspirational book of personal transformation and triumph. The narrative takes a different path, but it is—as Mewhorter suggested—his or her own way of describing their experience.

Since comic books are an excellent example of cancertainment and the way it navigates through the hazards of illness, I would like to focus instead on another form of popular culture—TV-series. I have chosen four such series, and I will present them shortly. I am aware that "Breaking Bad" is mentioned on many cancertainment lists, but in this case cancer serves as a catalyst rather than being an important part of the story as whole. I thus intend to focus instead on the following series: "The Big C," "Chasing Life," "New Amsterdam," and "Life Sentence."

"The Big C" aired from 2010 till 2013. The show follows Westhill High School teacher Cathy Jamison—who can be characterized as a reserved suburban wife and mother. She is diagnosed with stage IV melanoma. She decides that she doesn't want to share this information and burden her family and friends. So, she keeps it a secret for months. During this time, the only person she reveals her illness to is an elderly neighbor, Marlene, after the latter figures it out for herself, since her dog—Thomas, who spends a lot of time hanging around Cathy—can sniff out cancer. Cathy's behavior dramatically changes as she begins to make more and more foolhardy choices in the face of her approaching death. These include kicking her husband out of the house, spending money on an expensive car and having an affair. Thanks to these adventures, she unintentionally makes a bigger mess of her life and decides to put a stop to her reckless behavior. She ends the affair when she is exposed and allows her husband to move back in after finally revealing to him that she is sick. She also decides to undergo high-risk treatment because she now knows that she wants to live. Although the initial results are promising, the treatment proves unsuccessful. In season four, Cathy plans for her inevitable and imminent death. The series shows how the diagnosis of a terminal illness changes a person's life and how that person may react to the news. What kind of problems appear? How should we deal with such a diagnosis and (not) go crazy, how should we share this news with our family and friends, what decisions should we make regarding treatment and accepting support from others. The program also addresses the issues of what is truly important in life and what constitutes the essence of existence. While the main character may not be the best and realistic example of a cancer patient, she nevertheless confronts the main issues that shape the narratives of many cancer patients.

The second series—"Chasing Life"—aired for two seasons in 2014 and 2015 and is the American version of the Mexican television series "Terminales." It follows the life of 24-year-old April, who is an intelligent and ambitious young journalist trying to advance her career at a Boston newspaper. She is determined to impress her editor, but her illness derails her plans. April tries to balance her career aspirations with her family life. She lives with her widowed mom Sara, rebellious little sister Brenna, and her strong and generous grandmother. She is also involved romantically with Dominic, her co-worker. When she finds out from her estranged uncle that she has leukemia, her life falls apart, not simply because of the illness itself, but also because nobody seriously believes she has leukemia. When her editor asks her to write about cancer, she learns more about herself and her condition. The second person in this drama is Leo, the son of a famous politician, who is also a cancer patient. And as this is a love story, Leo falls for April and tries to win her heart. Eventually he asks her to marry him, she says "yes," and they get married. Shortly afterwards, he passes away in his sleep and April remains alone and cancer free, but afflicted with a sense of enormous loss. The story focuses on many things, the most important of which are the different stages that a terminally ill person must pass through in their struggle with cancer. Initially, nobody believes that her illness is anything serious, as her youth means she does not conform to the stereotype of a cancer patient. This is not how people imagine a cancer patient. April has to fight first to overcome the stereotype and then the stigma of cancer itself. The next stage in her struggle is the feeling that her body has betrayed her, that it is not even her body. Being brave enough to look at how her body has been ravaged by treatment is even worse than convincing people that she is ill. Her body image changes as the construction of her identity evolves. Furthermore, she must change her attitude as to what is truly important in life and dismiss what is driven purely by her ego. She must reevaluate her whole existence. She manages to overcome her cancer. She convinces Leo to fight his own illness. They overcome many obstacles, as Leo loses his memory following an operation. They both learn how to deal with life after cancer, which is another very important yet overlooked theme.

The above two TV-series were criticized for their lack of authentic characters, even though I felt April came across as quite convincing. There has been some debate as to the fact that these series have little in common with cancer in "real life" situations. The most important thing to bear in mind, however, was that an ill person, i.e. a cancer patient, does not look that nice. This is, I feel, the biggest issue with television, which, as Mary Valle also pointed out, tends to shows us pleasant looking, attractive blondes. And the hard truth is that after chemotherapy people look awful and they feel that way too. There is nothing sexy in a body destroyed by chemotherapy. But what many cancer patients forget to mention is that they also have a need to be loved and be beautiful. They need acceptance and support. That is also why some of the foundations working in this area use photography and characterization to give ill people a little break from the harsh everyday lives they lead.

The third television depiction of cancer takes place in a hospital headed by a new medical director Max Goodwin, who is also suffering from the disease. The series began in 2018 and is still airing. Max is very specific director—he breaks the rules to find a way to protect the unprotected by the system and to provide everyone with help. He adheres to a strict set of values, and because he is a workaholic he decides to undergo treatment while still working. All his struggles are visible to viewers, but he himself refuses to admit he has any problems with his health or that he needs assistance and support. His attitude changes when he meets a group of patients who spend their time during chemotherapy playing cards and fooling around. For example, in the 15th episode of the first season, they play a game in which they refer to their illnesses with joke names based on famous musicals—and thus "Mamma Mia" becomes Mamma Mastectomy, the "Fiddler on the Roof" becomes the Fiddler on the Puke and so on. Initially, Max is quite shocked by their jocularity and upbeat outlook on life. After all, surely they should be terrified by their cancer, their chemotherapy and the inevitability of death. But after a day of hardship, he begins to understand that it is through jokes and laughter that they can cope with everything that is thrown at them. It enables them to take control over part of their life, it helps them bond with each other. Some aspects of cancer shown in the show are perhaps not entirely realistic (working while undergoing treatment—even though I know a few people who tried to do the same thing), but the bonding effect and the use of joke names for cancer based on musicals are very realistic and helpful tools in real life. General views on cancer also appear to be changing as people use their natural coping mechanisms to deal with something as unimaginable as cancer.

Survivor Syndrome

There is one more cancer narrative that features in cancertainment productions, namely the stories of survivors. There are not many of them as the subject is mostly neglected. The CW series from 2017–2018 entitled "Life Sentence" best encapsulates this theme. This is the story of a young female suffering from terminal cancer. She has been ill for most of her life and that is why her whole family has done everything they can to make her limited time on earth as happy as possible. Stella Abbott—the main character—benefits from experimental treatment. As nothing had worked in the past she had for most of her life been given little chance of reaching her twenties. But now she needs to learn how to really live. Her and her family's attitude was "to live like she was going to die the very next day." As they learn that she will be able to lead a cancer-free life, they have to face all the consequences of the lies and destructive decisions they have made over the years. After all, they had thought their sister and daughter would die. She and her husband have to survive the struggle too, as now they have to create a real life for themselves, not a fake one which had been adapted solely to her needs. Stella's post-cancer life seems to be even harder than when she was a patient. Stella has no education, no job experience, no real friends. Her family is falling apart and her marriage is not real either. The opportunity of a cancer-free life—which should have been a miracle—has turned out to be more disastrous than her previous existence as an ill person.

The series was cancelled after one season as some viewers were outraged at the very idea that health itself could be treated as a problem. However, the struggle is real and some studies show that following remission from cancer many people have problems fitting into the life they have been given. Life for such people seemed easier when they were cancer patients, because they were familiar with this role, than when as cancer survivors they were expected to adjust to a new reality—they are no longer the same person they were before they had cancer. They cannot come back to their previous lives and they must rediscover their identities on a new path and as a new self. The shock and stress caused by the prospect of having a "long life" ahead of them is very real.

Anette L. Stanton, Julienne E. Bower and Carissa A. Low see in this kind of situation the possibility of posttraumatic growth. In their opinion "some cancer patients report profound positive changes in themselves, their relationships, and other life domains after cancer." They focus on patients who reported "enhanced interpersonal relationships, a greater appreciation for life, sense of increased personal strength, greater spirituality, and valued change in life priorities or goals" (Stanton et al. 2006, pp. 140–141). Brad J. Zebrack points out that with a cancer diagnosis comes a change in the way one sees one's self. Most research has focused on the change initiated by the cancer diagnosis itself, which is widely known and recognized in the literature. This shift in attitude allows cancer survivors to value life more. It also "involves changes in social roles and identity" (Zebrack 2001, p. 238). However, the transformation that results from fighting cancer is also a cause of distress as it opens up new possibilities. On the other hand, cancer survivors never rid themselves of the feeling that their illness is gone for good. However, this distress may be due to many factors (Aaronson et al. 2014).

Does it work and for whom?

Some campaigns share the testimonies of cancer patients, which highlight many issues. One woman, who had breast cancer, wrote (bolded fragments by Ł.L.):

> Be aware of this: **the culture of breast cancer has created a schism among women with the disease**. [...] Women with early-stage disease are actively encouraged to tout all they have DONE to FIGHT and BEAT **a disease that has nothing if not randomness on its side**. We are only **supposed to be bald once, to go through treatment once**. We are **not supposed to bother the world with having cancer for the rest of our lives**. The culture tells us this is TIRING. The culture encourages women with lazy or passive cancer to feel superior to women with brutal and aggressive cancer. But **we are all living in bodies where something went wrong. Nobody wins"** (Ennis-O'Connor 2015).

The "culture of cancer" stands somewhat in opposition to cancertainment. It generates opinions and views on cancer, on its causes, on how people should behave, on the nature and types of treatment, on what kind of cancer is "normal" for whom and so on. Melba Newsome (2008) wrote in an article about young women with cancer that in many cases their illness had been misdiagnosed because they were thought to be "too young for cancer."

> Jen is a member of the disease's orphan generation—young adults left behind in the age of research and increasing survival rates. Because they and their doctors ignore signs that would scream "cancer" in someone older, they often go months without a proper diagnosis. What is worse, when some types of cancer are discovered, they tend to be the types that spread aggressively to other parts of the body, offering a slimmer chance of survival (Newsome 2008).

On the one hand, the "culture of cancer" tends to give a false sense of security, while on the other it envisages treatment in terms of a "battle" or a "war." If you lose, if you don't put up a fight, you should feel ashamed. Cancertainment exposes the harsh truth of cancer but does so in an ironic, satiric and sometimes even sarcastic way. It shifts from a "this is war" point of view to a more honest, emotional and broader way of seeing oneself. It focuses on the body—how we feel it, how it betrays us, how it falls apart, and how it tries to recover. It sees the importance of interactions—between patients and doctors, between cancer patients and other people, between family members and between friends. Most of all, it focuses on knowledge about different types of cancer, available treatments, side effects and the ugly truth about each aspect and each stage of life with cancer.

Heidi Schultz Adams and Christopher Schultz (2010) highlighted seven aspects of the life of a cancer patient: the diagnosis, dealing with the diagnosis, the treatment, the side effects, the mental state of the patient, interactions with people and life after cancer. In all these areas cancertainment can provide us with information, and at the same time simply make us laugh and relax a little, which is the most welcome reaction. Some of those diagnosed with cancer feel that joking about their condition was their way of coping. However, such people had tended to have rather sarcastic personalities even in their pre-cancer lives, hence such attitudes are typical for some and may not be helpful for others. In an interview with "Newsweek," Iva Skoch told Rebecca Shabad (2009) that she found it natural to see all the absurdities and odd things that a young person would. She also said:

> I also feel, like a lot of survivors I talked to, in so many ways, cancer was the best thing that ever happened to me just because it puts such a different perspective on your life. Cancer, the word, does not scare me anymore; it used to. If somebody says "I have cancer," cancer is a thousand different diseases. It's not one disease. I try not to use it as a blanket statement for anything anymore because I think that word carries such a stigma (Skoch and Shabad 2009).

Christine Clifford (Schoenberg 2012) also tried to seek "humor in her tumor," claiming that "My whole push has been, let's help cancer patients get back into the mainstream of life, and I think humor is a great way to do that. It makes you feel like your life is normal." In turn, Nara Schoenberg (2012) observed that: "due in part to declining cancer death rates, an increase in the number of support groups and the breast cancer movement, all of which have brought survivors together and affirmed their experiences, along with factors such as increasing openness in both society and comedy, cancer humor—long an unofficial part of the patient experience—is coming out of the closet." The more coverage there is about cancer—in books, films, TV-shows, etc.—the more chances those confronting a cancer diagnosis will have to find their own ways of coping with their lot.

In an article on the topic of cancertainment on screen Anne Moyer and Jackelyn Payne (2018) argued that: "Given the growing number of cancer survivors, more accurately portraying the average experience of cancer could provide a great benefit to those experiencing cancer in real life." They also believe that it is important to study the influence of TV-shows on cancer patients and their moods, as we still have limited knowledge of "bibliotherapy" and the "use of narratives in the form of books." In their opinion:

> If it helps individuals process their experiences, or if it will help loved ones or caregivers understand some of what the patient or survivor is going through, then, by all means, they should bust out the popcorn. But it's important to take it with a grain (or sprinkle) of salt. Survival rates for many types of cancer are improving, and different people experience it in different ways. Above all, it's important for patients to remember that a cancer diagnosis doesn't define them, which is an idea often perpetuated by Hollywood and the film industry in general. Real people are not plot points meant to move storylines along (Moyer, Payne 2018).

In my opinion, this approach works for all of us who like to be open and helpful. It may help those who suffer and those who need support. It is a useful tool for creating positive memories from the far from positive experience of illness. But it also requires a critical evaluation, as the attitudes to cancer may differ, because they are individual and unique. Also, how a person reacts to treatment and their odds of beating it vary greatly from individual to individual, as Moyer and Payne pointed out. Such diverging experiences must be taken into account when trying to gauge the influence of pop culture in raising awareness about cancer and the therapeutical role of films and TV-series.

Conclusions

The TV representations of cancer presented above were discussed and compared with personal experiences—online forums have provided tv-show producers with valuable insights on how to create more vivid and authentic characters and plots. Hence, comments made by cancer patients could be used to modify even characters deemed to be insufficiently realistic. Such shows help us talk about our own illness, by discussing the stories people watch, read or listen to. Another thing is that adopting a humorous stance on illness may serve a cleansing role, not only by helping patients and their loved ones cope with better understand their situation and bond with others but also as a means of breaking the ice when talking with non-cancer people, who are afraid how to behave and what to say. By joking about one's own cancer they can open up the conversation. We can learn a great deal from these products of pop culture and gain a greater understanding of the predicament of the cancer patient.

Cartoons, movies, books and other such media help the cancer patient realize they are not alone. Moreover, playing, reading and writing help clear the mind and reduce anxiety, shift the patient's interest elsewhere and focus on things that appear more manageable at that very moment. Most importantly, however, it enables the patient to maintain their dignity, overcome their feelings of powerlessness, and instill a belief that the cancer can be beaten. A person who actively confronts their cancer by making jokes about it and writing accounts of their experience claims ownership over their story and reclaims power over their body and their illness. Cancertainment may not remove the stigma hanging over cancer, but it can help sufferers and their loved ones cope with the negative connotations of "cancer culture." It certainly makes a difference, which should be the subject of more precise research.

References

Aaronson N.K., Mattioli V., Minton O., Weis J., Johansen C., Dalton S.O., Verdonck de Leeuw I.M., Stein K.D., Alfano C.M., Mehnert A., de Boer A. 2014. Beyond treatment—psychological and behavioural issues in cancer survivorship research and practice. *European Journal of Cancer Supplements* 12(1): 54–64.

Cancer Schamcer Movement. *Our Mission*. Available at: https://www.cancerschmancer.org/our-mission. Accessed: 20.04.2021.

Engleberg M. 2006. *Cancer Made Me A Shallower Person: A Memoir in Comics*. New York: Harper Collins.

Ennis-O'Connor M. 2015. Weekly round up: Stomp out breast cancer edition. *Journeying Beyond Breast Cancer. Making Sense of the Breast Cancer Experience Together*, March 8. Available at: https://journeyingbeyondbreastcancer.com/2015/03/08/weekly-round-up-96-2/. Accessed: 22.04.2021.

FreakCitySF. 2009. *Cancertainment. Urban Dictionary*. Available at: https://www.urbandictionary.com/define.php?term=cancertainment. Accessed: 22.04.2021.

IARC, International Agency for Research on Cancer. 2018. Cancer Today. *Global Cancer Observatory*. Available at: https://gco.iarc.fr/today/online-analysis-map?v=2018. Accessed: 22.04.2021.

Jowsa A. 2019. *Wystawa „Choroba jako źródło sztuki" w Muzeum Narodowym w Poznaniu*. Dzieje.pl. April 28. Available at: https://dzieje.pl/wystawy/wystawa-choroba-jako-zrodlo-sztuki-w-muzeum-narodowym-w-poznaniu. Accessed: 22.04.2021.

Kozyra K. 1996. *Olympia* (video installation). Available at: https://zacheta.art.pl/pl/kolekcja/katalog/kozyra-katarzyna-olimpia. Accessed: 22.04.2021.

Mewhorter M. *Cancer Owl*. Available at: https://cancerowl.com/. Accessed: 22.04.2021.

Mewhorter M. 2015. Cancer, comics, and having the guts to talk about it. *Lacuna Loft*, October 21. Available at: https://lacunaloft.org/cancer-comics-guts-talk/. Accessed: 22.04.2021.

Moyer A., Payne J. 2018. Cancer on screen as "cancertainment." *Psychology Today*. November 16. Available at: https://www.psychologytoday.com/ie/blog/beyond-treatment/201811/cancer-screen-cancertainment. Accessed: 22.04.2021.

Newsome M. 2008. Young women living with cancer. *Women's Health. Online magazine*. November 3. Available at: https://www.womenshealthmag.com/sex-and-love/a19928444/cancer-questions-answered/. Accessed: 22.04.2021.
Planet Cancer. *Cancertainment*. Available at: http://64.62.179.30/html/cancertainment.php?sec_Id=2. Accessed: 22.04.2021.
Scambler G., Scambler S. 2010. *New Directions in the Sociology of Chronic and Disabling Conditions. Assaults on the Lifeworld*. New York: Palgrave Macmillian.
Schoenberg N. 2012. Cancer's funny? *Chicago Tribune*, November 16. Available at: https://www.chicagotribune.com/lifestyles/health/sc-health-1107-cancer-humor-20121107-story.html. Accessed: 21.04.2021.
Schultz Adams D.H. 2008. Planet cancer: A community of young adults with cancer. *Journal of Oncology Practice* 4(4): 189.
Schultz Adams D.H., Schultz C. 2010. *Planet Cancer. The Frequently Bizarre Yet Always Informative Experiences and Thoughts of Your Fellow Natives*. Lyons Press.
Skoch I., Rosenthal K. 2009. Young people living, and laughing, with cancer. *NPR: Fresh Air*. September 8. Available at: https://www.npr.org/templates/story/story.php?storyId=112563650&t=1604881125295. Accessed: 22.04.2021.
Skoch I., Shabad R. 2009. QA: Iva Skoch on cancertainment. *Newsweek*. July 31. Available at: https://www.newsweek.com/qa-iva-skoch-cancertainment-222576. Accessed: 22.04.2021.
Stanton A.L., Bower J.E., Low C.A. 2006. Posttraumatic growth after cancer. In *Handbook of Posttraumatic Growth. Research and Practice*, eds. L.G. Calhoun, R.G. Tedeschi, 138–175. New York–London: Psychology Press Taylor and Francis.
Szabo L. 2006. Laughing in the face of cancer. *USA Today*. May 23. Available at: https://usatoday30.usatoday.com/life/books/news/2006-05-22-cancer-comics_x.htm. Accessed: 22.04.2021.
Triage Cancer. *Haidi Adams*. Available at: https://triagecancer.org/heidi-adams. Accessed: 22.04.2021.
Valle M. 2010. That's cancertainment! *Killing the Buddha*. October 18. Available at: https://killingthebuddha.com/mag/confession/thats-cancertainment/. Accessed: 22.04.2021.
WHO, World Health Organization 2021. *Cancer*. Available at: https://www.who.int/health-topics/cancer. Accessed: 22.04.2021.
Zebrack B.J. 2001. Cancer Survivor Identity and Quality of Life. *Cancer Practice* 8(5): 238–242.

Barbara Bojdo

Style and Ideological Changes in Depicting Death in European Art from Roman Antiquity to the Renaissance

Abstract

Particularly interesting aspect of iconography in European art beginning from antiquity to modern times is depiction of death. The subject of this paper will mainly be focused on iconographic themes associated with it, like representations of mortality in antiquity including architectural forms such as mausoleums and iconographic programs sculpted on the Roman sarcophagi (I BC–IV AD). There will be also presented works of art in which the significance of death was presented in a religious context, such as iconographic programs from decorative portals from the Romanesque period as well as tombstone monuments in transi (cadaver) type which spread all over the Europe in the art of late Middle Ages (late 14th–16th c.). Works of art will be discussed in relation to their function and also in reference to the iconographic program contained therein. Furthermore, in the paper will be shown the socio-cultural aspect, which is fundamental for depicting death in discussed periods, with particular emphasis on maxims: *Memento Mori* and *Vanitas vanitatum et omnia vanitas.* In the reflection on the depiction of passing away beginning from the Romanesque period the particular emphasis will be placed on the issue of the prevalence of the Last Judgment and Purgatory representations. The paper will also analyze the question of whether the presented image of the passing away in past periods may have or even has a reference to modern times.

Keywords: death, Last Judgment, Purgatory, transi tombs, passing away

Vita brevis breviter in brevi finietur,
mors venit velociter quae neminem veretur,
omnia mors perimit et nulli miseretur.
Et nulli miseretur.[1]

Introduction

A special aspect in art is the theme of depicting death. This iconographic motif appears in art from antiquity to modern times. Beginning from the great civilizations such as the civilizations of ancient Rome through the Middle Ages until present times, both in the literature and in the visual arts various depictions of death frequently appear. The image itself is not always isolated in the form of a specific work of art, or a specific sculptural representation but it is quite often part of huge religious representation like in the Romanesque portals or like in total work of art where comes to harmonious synthesis of architectural, sculptural or painting masterpieces such as grave complexes or entire funeral assumptions proper to given era such as Roman remains from Glanum in France (c. 40 AD), *Campo Santo* in Pisa (13th c.), *Certosa* in Bologna (14th c.) or established in the beginning of 19th century *Cimitero Monumentale* in Milan. Motifs showing passing away, which are appearing in imaging and symbolism, become very clearly visible mostly when an artistic expression is combined with ideology, tradition and also when they are connected with the spheres of *sacrum* and *profanum*. Looking at the "deadly" images beginning from those that have become established in the Roman Empire through the phenomenon of funeral art of the Middle Ages, we can learn about the development and changes in their meaning and in some sense also about the function of burial itself.

Individual death, and thus the thought of the coming end, is constantly present in European culture and art. However, depending on an epoch, this imaging had a different dimension and also a different background. In Roman times, Imperial death imagery was highly secularized, and the burial itself was quite propagandist. Changes have come along with the development of the art of so-called early Christianity art. References to propaganda have been supplanted by burial traditions combined with religious reflection. The passing away becomes an unmodified part of the existence of a human being,

[1] "Life is short, and shortly it will end; Death comes quickly and respects no one, Death destroys everything and takes pity on no one. To death we are hastening, let us refrain from sinning" (*Ad Mortem Festinămus*, Llibre Vermell de Montserrat 1399).

and the awareness of the upcoming death includes knowledge about the limitation of being, and the inevitable end.

Depicting of death in European art from Roman antiquity to the Renaissance

In the culture of Rome, funeral performances were something more than just devotional objects, they were also a very helpful medium in spreading political and religious beliefs throughout the Roman Empire. For example, tombs and funeral complexes, such as mausoleums[2] (Figs. 1 and 2), were *memoriae* for the deceased, commemorating the dead one through the dimensions of the building itself, as well as self-presentation inscriptions.[3] The goal of mentioned *memoriae* (Fig. 3) was to emphasize the greatness of the actions of the deceased, both immediately after his death and many centuries later, where we have an opportunity to study, admire or criticize their attitude, just like the ancients right after the death of the individuals. However, whether it was immediately after the death of the commemorated person or at present times the message that this type of burial carried with him was and still is legible: commemorating the deceased and emphasized the propaganda dimension by giving the opportunity of constant experience of Imperial greatness and eternity preserved sometimes in written word but certainly in the monumental tombstones, which highlighted the achievements, deeds and ambitions of the deceased (Davies 2000).

An especially important group of monuments of origins from *Imperium Romanum* which have a funeral character are sarcophagi. On sarcophagi mostly from the 2nd–3rd centuries and initially also in the 4th century were decorated by figural decorations in relief with motifs such as battle scenes (Fig. 4), hunting scenes (Fig. 5) and also biographical scenes including episodes from the life of the deceased including their portraits (Fig. 6). The second group of sarcophagi are those on which mythological scenes were depicted (Fig. 7). These scenes are often analogous to those chosen for the decoration of private spaces, such as the interiors of houses, however in sepulchral art in most cases they acquire a different meaning. Some researchers believe that the scenes depicted on the sarcophagi have purely symbolic significance

[2] Examples of mausoleums preserved *in situ*: Mausoleum of the Julii from Glanum (France); Rome—Mausoleum of Emperor Hadrian (Castel Sant'Angelo) and Mausoleum of Emperor Augustus, Fabara (Spain)—Mausoleum of Lucius Aemilius Lupus.

[3] Copy of edited in 1938. *Res Gestae Divi Augusti* (*Memoriae* of Emperor Augustus in form of inscription), is carved and filled with bronze letters on the exterior wall of the Museum of the *Ara Pacis* in Rome (Rossini 2009).

related to the religious beliefs of the Romans regarding death and life after death. In turn, another research trend underlines that the choice of classical iconography is only intended to accentuate the sublimity of classical culture, and thus to show the deceased as its connoisseur, which was to emphasize or increase the status of the deceased (Avan 2000). The use of sarcophagi for burials lasted until the Christian period, in which they became an important medium conveying the ideology of the new religion. With the appearance of early Christian funerary art representations associated with the Emperor and the Empire disappear. This new ideology brings changes in sculptural decorations shown on the sarcophagi (Fig. 8), their current subject matter has been related to Christian wisdom and to the contemplation of truths revealed in the Old and New Testaments (Evans 1993, pp. 77–84). The iconography currently presented in the near future would forever ousted classical iconography and survived in the history of art as Christian art.

Monumental manifestation of depiction of death in Christian iconography are representations of the Last Judgments. This motif appears primarily in portal sculpture of French Romanesque art in the 12th century. As life in the Middle Ages is inseparable bond with the ubiquitous death which is manifested in the short life of the average citizen of that times, in the deaths of infants and mothers in the puerperium, or in omnipresent diseases and widespread plagues, the imaging of death becomes an inherent iconographic motif of that era. Following the famous medieval sentence *Memento Mori* in the art of the Middle Ages, especially in the Last Judgments, the image of death was immortalized as pervasive, inevitable and being a constant component of the earthly life of contemporary man. In the Romanesque Last Judgments the death was shown as a phenomenon that does not clearly mean the end of human life. With this type of imaging, only the earthly existence is completed, and the path continues in the afterlife. In connection with the doctrine of two worlds functioning in the Middle Ages, everyone was troubled by the question of where would lead the last path, would the individual one be able to reach the land of full grace which is heaven or would be thrown into hell, where would be condemned to perpetual torment (Brooks 1989)? Romanesque artists wonderfully showed this dualistic picture of the afterlife world in frieze from Lincoln Cathedral (Fig. 9)—circa 1140 (Maher et al. 2000, p. 225) and tympanums of Baulieu-sur-Dordogne (Fig. 10)—c. 1130/c. 1135, Conques-en-Rouergue (Fig. 11)—c. 1130/c. 1140, and also in Autun (Fig 12.)—after 1125 (Hearn 1985, pp. 178–183). On the frieze we may see four panels with damned accompanied by demons and devils which are preceding one and the most significant panel with depiction of mouth of hell with sinners swallowed to knock them down in to the hellish abyss, with some of the damned saved by Christ, which is trampling the demon (Fig. 9).[4] In all of the iconographic programs depicted in tympanums, enthroned Christ is shown on the axis of the portal. Mentioned two words are depicted: in case of Baulieu the tympanum is divided into the upper and lower registers: heaven and hell, in the two other portals the scenes form tympanums take places on the right and left side of enthroned Christ. The vision of heaven does not cause any concerns, it is idyllic and optimistic, however the Romanesque depiction of hell is not a nice and pleasant vision. The vision of apocalyptic animals from Baulieu (Fig. 13), demons and devil separating punishments in Conques (Figs. 14 and 15) and devils and monstrous creatures brewing souls in Autun (Figs. 16 and 17) probably had tremendous power of influence on everyone who entered the temple under the portal, because every single contemporary man ware aware with *Biblia Pauperum* and according to that knowledge can easily recognized all sins, and thus was conscious to which kingdom the lifetime could be leading (Jelonek 2002). It is also worth to mention a great example of Last Judgment from Florence Baptistery of Saint John from 13th century, immortalized in the mosaic, with iconographic program similar to those from the French Romanesque tympanums with representations of dualistic world and enthroned Christ (Figs. 18 and 19). The heavenly kingdom is depicted on the right sight of enthroned Christ, and hellish abyss with all kinds of demons, devils and monstrous creatures are shown on His left (Giusti 2000, pp. 72–75).

In Gothic, the Last Judgments are still portrayed for example in the portals of great 13th century cathedrals like in Bourges—Saint-Étienne Cathedral (Figs. 20 and 21) and in Paris—Notre Dame Cathedral (Figs. 22 and 23). But we have also other representations of death such as Crucifixions (Fig. 24), so called *Vesperbilder* or *Pietà* sculptures[5] (Fig. 25) or tombstones showing the full figurative realistic portrait of the deceased—the *gisant* tombstone (Fig. 26).

Vanitas vanitatum et omnia vanitas[6]—transi as a body image, of an individual who has passed away. An image in innovative form which refers to the decay, loss of worldly goods, turning into dust and the disappearance of corporality, which appears in funeral art in the end of 14th century. Transi tombs in their vanity show what was before hidden under the flesh, robe or

[4] Similar and also contemporary depiction of Hellmouth was painted in Winchester Psalter, an illuminated manuscript from XII century (British Library collection). Available at: http://www.bl.uk/manuscripts/Viewer.aspx?ref=cotton_ms_nero_c_iv_f039r. Accessed: 10.11.2020.

[5] Depiction of the seated Virgin Mary with the body of a dead Christ on her lap. The genesis of this iconographic motif can be traced on the examples of 13th century sculptures from Germany through 14th century examples from the Czech Republic and Poland, finishing on Italian origins masterpieces from the turn of the 15th and 16th centuries sculpted by Michelangelo (Kalinowski 1953, pp. 20–34).

[6] Vanity of vanities and all is vanity (own translation).

an armor in classical gisant tombs (Fig. 26). Transi emphasizes the fact that after death an individual one loses his temporal identity by transforming the body into a corpse, in turn a corpse into a skeleton, and the portrait itself is a picture not of the deceased one but of the signs of death (Fig. 27). If in the early Middle Ages we had mainly iconographic references to the Last Judgment and an emanation of human feelings should to be a fear of soul brewing, that in the late Middle Ages in imaging of ultimate matters, depiction of Purgatory become widespread (Mirsanu 2008, pp. 179–193).[7] Simultaneously with wide spreading of purgatory doctrine a new phenomenon appears in the form of gravestones. Cadaver tombs or transi (from French word which means "passed over") are sculptural depictions of an anatomical image of the body at various stages of decay.

From my research work it is quite evident that amongst almost all cadaver type graves representation, few of them are curved in very good anatomical manner. It would seem that Leonardo da Vinci was the precursor of the anatomical image of the human body (Fig. 28) in the process of synergy between science and art (Keele and Roberts 1983). However, in the analysis of transi-type tombs from the 14th-16th centuries, we can certainly conclude that the anatomical image of the human body was also known to medieval sculptors. Examples of this phenomenon are only few, but its existence cannot be denied. Analyzing the sculpture workshop of transi type graves, especially those located *in situ* in churches and cathedrals of England, we can indicate that the sculptors which carved the effigy tombstones were familiar with human anatomy. The anatomical details that can be indicated on the cadaver tombstones were made with such precision, that it could be concluded without any hesitation, that they were made by people who experienced death and deadness, just like modernly a practitioner in the field of forensic medicine. These specific mortality images are an indication of all signs of decay. Sometimes they are only depicted by dried corpses, on which under the thin layer of skin can be seen tendons, ribs, veins or sagging cheeks that emphasize sharpness of facial features fantastically visible in sculpture from transi tombs such as 15th century cadavers of: Archbishop Henry Chichele from Canterbury (Figs. 29 and 30), Alice de la Pole from Ewelme (Figs. 31 and 32), Bishop Thomas Beckington from Wells (Figs. 33 and 34) and also of Cardinal Jean de la Grange from Avignon (Fig. 35). An another example of deadly image is a picture of a rotting body, in a terminal state of decay with worms crawling out of the eye sockets or open cavities in the body which we may analyze on an example of cadaver tomb—*l'homme à moulons* from La Chapelle Funérai-

[7] Purgatory matter appears in Latin Church dogma since the Second Council of Lyon (1274).

re des Seigneurs de Boussu in Belgium (16th c.).[8] The decomposition stadium in which the rotting process began, we can also analyze based on a great example of full figure 16th century sculpture of Jeanne de Burbon-Vendôme (Figs. 36 and 37). Analyzing the phenomenon of monuments in the transi type, it can be assumed that showing the body in a various states of decay was aimed at establishing a dialogue between the viewer and the image. Perhaps the deceased needed some help on the soul's journey through purgatory, and the attempt to show the decaying body was to help the individual by arousing the viewer's need to say a prayer for him? On confirming the advisability of correspondence between the transi and the viewer is an inscription engraved on the cadaver tomb from Avignon: Spectaculum facti sumus mundo, ut maior[res et] minores, in nobis clare [per]uidant, ad quem statum redigentur, nemin[en ex]cipiendo, cuiusuis sta[tu]s, / sexus uel etatis. ergo miser cur superbi[s n]am cinis es, et in cadauer fetidum, cibum et escam vermium, ac cinerem sic et nos, reverter which briefly means:

> We have been made a spectacle for the world so that the older and the younger may look clearly upon us, in order that they might see to what state they will be reduced. No one is excluded, regardless of estate, sex, or age. Therefore, miserable one, why are you proud? You are only ash, and you will revert, as we have done to a fetid cadaver, food and tidbits for worms, and ashes (Cohen 1973, pp. 103–104).

The procedure of showing the difference between wet—corporal and dry—skeletonal stage of body decomposition was able to serve as a visual tool aimed at stimulating the imagination of living viewers in order to show that they can also go to purgatory post-mortem, and therefore that they should to take care of their souls already in the life time (Welch 2013, pp. 133–155). Vision of the afterlife in the late medieval period is strictly connected with the theological vision of purgatory with all of the pain, suffering and doubts filling this sphere. We should be certain that former viewers never dare to underestimate the traditional, cultural and devotional division of the underworld. Even Dante in his *La Divina Commedia*[9] depicted the passage through three spheres of underworld: hell, purgatory and heaven (Fig. 38). This dramatically illustrated passage firstly in Dante's masterpiece, then immortalized in the Botticelli's paintings, shows a cross-section of all of the punishments which was waiting for the sinner (Parker 2013, pp. 84–102). This imaginary from cadaver tombs, from Dante's *La Divina Commedia* and also from Botticelli's *Inferno*[10] may have quite an educational dimension especially in that

---

[8] Images of Boussu cadaver: Available at: https://chateaudeboussu.be/decouvrir/la-chapelle-funeraire. Accessed: 10.11.2020.

[9] Poem written by Dante in c. 1308–1320. First printed edition was published in 1472.

[10] Images of Botticelli's Inferno c. 1485: *La mappa dell'inferno* (Chart of Hell)—page 101R: Available at: https://digi.vatlib.it/view/MSS_Reg.lat.1896.pt.A Sinners in torment—detail form

specific period of time. For medieval viewers that kind representation could be some kind of warning or even a incentive to make a prayer to avoid some of tremendous punishments in the way thru afterlife, but it could be also helpful to the decay one, if he meant to go to purgatory in his afterlife, because by the prayers the punishment may become lesser. No matter the needs of an author or the founder of cadaver tomb was, the main and most important dimension of its uprising is the fact that its significance and the message carried by that kind of imaginary was predicted to less-educated members of late medieval society. It's the same medium as *Biblia Pauperum* in the early medieval period, but now speaks by the corpses—naked, even humiliated, humble in death but full of educational power. Those corpses became to be the socio-cultural media gave by religious, clerical or medieval establishments to the rest of medieval society, probably to achieve a double gain by giving some kind of hope to the other sinners and also for themselves by making lesser punishment if they went to purgatory in their afterlife way. However, in the case of transi tombstones, not only the vision of the salvation of the soul in purgatory plays a role in their dissemination over two centuries. The black death epidemic (Bridbury 1973) and the so-called great famine (Jordan 1997), which flooded Europe in the 14th century, could also become the basis for showing the vanity of the human body. The tradition of showing the body post-mortem remained in sepulchral art until the 16th century, where examples of this type of tombs are two royal burial groups from Cathedral of St. Denis—tomb of Louis XII and Anne of Bretagne and the tomb of Henry II and Catherine de'Medici (Bass 2017). Mentioned tombs are constructed in the form of two-level foundation, where the transi of the royal couple are located on the catafalque, and above them at the crowning level of the tomb are disposed full-figure, realistic sculptures of the royals (Figs. 39 and 40). In case of the 16th century cadaver tombs from St. Denis an image of body post-mortem is serene, delicate and sublime, with no visible signs of decomposition (Figs. 41 and 42). According to cadaver tombs from 15th century, we are also dealing with two-level foundations (Fig. 43), however, the transi sculpted in previously discussed tombs, in my opinion, have much stronger visual and emotional impression on the contemporary recipient, due to the strong means of expression, which is the purpose of showing the human body in terminal stage of decomposition, so fantastically describe by simple sentence written by Michael Camille: *embodied in a static image the process of becoming nothing* (Camille 1996, p. 176).

Chart of Hel—page 99R: Available at: https://digi.vatlib.it/view/MSS_Reg.lat.1896.pt.A. Accessed: 10.11.2020.

Conclusions

The complexity of life and death as well as memory and forgetfulness has been recorded in the sepulchral art of all the epochs mentioned in the paper. However, in Roman antiquity, sepulchral sculpture takes forms that show the ideal state of the body and the soul united with it. In that period of time the body's purpose was to depict the idea not the temporality, with its changes, the time laps and final destruction. On the other hand, in medieval art, the image of a body devoid of soul is spreading. Whether in the representations of the Last Judgments of the 12th century or in case of widely discussed tombs in the type of transi, the deadness of the body is complete, and therefore temporality is the key issue here, and the awareness that the soul has already escaped from the body is the quintessence of the meaning of this type of representations in the socio-cultural context of an epoch. The fascination in passing away is tantamount to the sum of fear and curiosity that arouses in man the terminal state. From antiquity to modern times, this fear is unchangeable, psychologically, traditionally or sociologically conditioned, because we are aware that we are only fragile beings that do not know the day of the final judgment. These short descriptions may be quite accurate references also to the current situation with the pandemic of COVID-19. In past epochs people were aware of plagues and with the rumbling what they were carrying with themselves. The death so strictly connected with plagues was something inevitable, terrifying, reaching everyone, regardless of the status, position or possessed goods. Likewise in the present day, the virus also does not choose, it can reach everyone, however today we do not refer our fears of the finality to the macabre representations of death but to the statistics and first of all to the opinions of experts.

As a conclusion to this paper, I would like to cite a fragment of a poem which may perfectly illustrate decomposition of the human body post-mortem. This excerpt comes from a poem "The death of Słowacki" written by Polish poet Julian Tuwim, printed in 1929 in a book of poems entitled *Rzecz Czarnoleska*. That poem was written to commemorate another great Polish writer Juliusz Słowacki right after his death:

"Body? By caries decayed,
Body for ash grated
Palpitate in a black casket.
Not much of it, not much
Skull, withered crossbones ..."[11]

[11] Own translation from the Polish original.

References

Avan H.T. 2000. Roman Sarcophagy. In *Heilbrunn Timeline of Art History*. New York: The Metropolitan Museum of Art.

Bass M.A. 2017. The transi tomb and the genius of sixteenth-century Netherlandish funerary sculpture. *Netherlands Yearbook for History of Art* 67(1): 160–187.

Bridbury A.R. 1973. The black death. *The Economic History Review* 26(4): 577–592.

Brooks B.H. 1989. Religion, afterlife, and property rights in the high middle ages. *Studies in Economic Analysis* 12(1): 2–21.

Camille M. 1996. *Master of Death: The Lifeless Art of Pierre Remiet illuminator*, London: Yale University Press.

Cohen K. 1973. *Metamorphosis of a Death Symbol: The Transi Tomb in the Late Middle Ages and the Renaissance*, California: University Press.

Davies P.J.E. 2000. *Death and the Emperor. Roman Imperial Funerary Monuments from Augustus to Marcus Aurelius*. Cambridge: Cambridge University Press.

Evans H. 1993. An early Christian sarcophagus from Rome lost and found. *Metropolitan Museum Journal* 28: 77–84.

Hearn M.F. 1985. *Romanesque Sculpture*. New York: Cornell University Press.

Giusti A. 2000. *The Baptistery of San Giovanni in Florence*. Firenze: La Mandragora.

Jelonek T. 2002. Biblia pauperum „katechezą w średniowieczu." *Ruch Biblijny i Liturgiczny* 1–4: 16–21.

Jordan W. 1997. *The Great Famine*. New Jersey: Princeton University Press.

Kalinowski L. 1953. Geneza Piety Średniowiecznej. *Polska Akademia Umiejętności – Prace Komisji Historii Sztuki* X: 20–34.

Kelle K.D., Roberts J. 1983. *Leonardo da Vinci: Anatomical Drawings from the Royal Library, Windsor Castle*. New York: The Metropolitan Museum of Art.

Maher L., Borradaile G., Stewart J.D., O'Connor M. 2000. The Romanesque Frieze at Lincoln Cathedral (England)—primary or secondary insertion? Magnetic considerations. *Archncornefry* 42(I): 225–236.

Mirsanu D.G. 2008. Dawning awareness of the theology of purgatory in the East: A review. *Bucharest* 4(4): 179–193.

Parker D. 2013. Illuminating Botticelli's Chart of Hell. *MLN* 128(1), *Italian Issue*: 84–102.

Rossini O. 2009. *Res Gestae Divi Augusti*. Roma: Gangemi.

Welch C. 2013. For prayers and pedagogy: Contextualizing English Carved Cadaver Monuments of the late medieval social and religious elite. *Fieldwork in Religion* 8(2): 133–155.

Figures captions

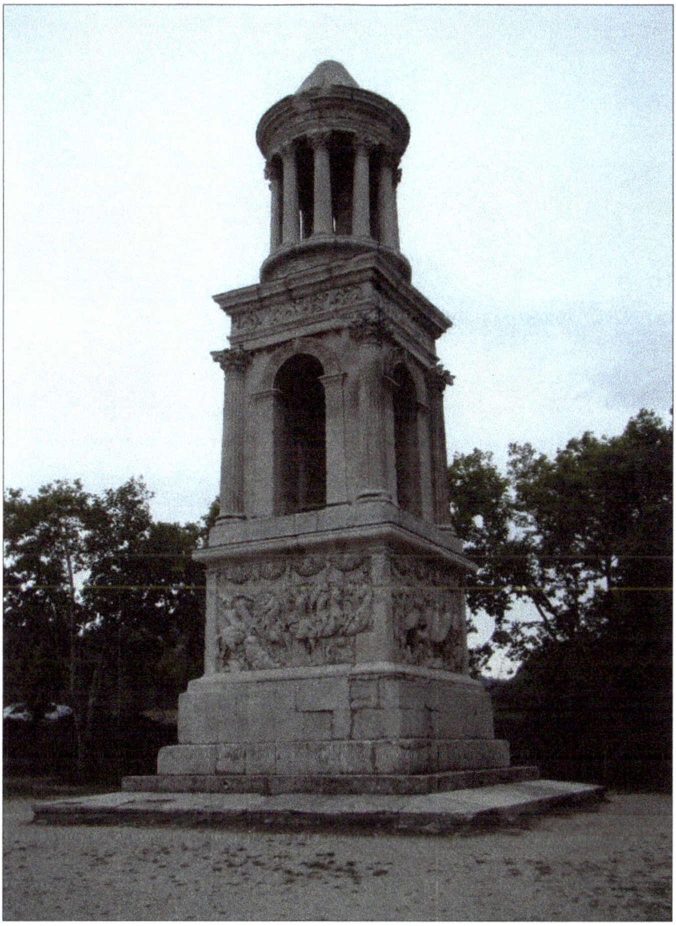

Figure 1. *Mausoleum of the Julii* (c. 40 BC), Glanum, Barbara Bojdo (2012)

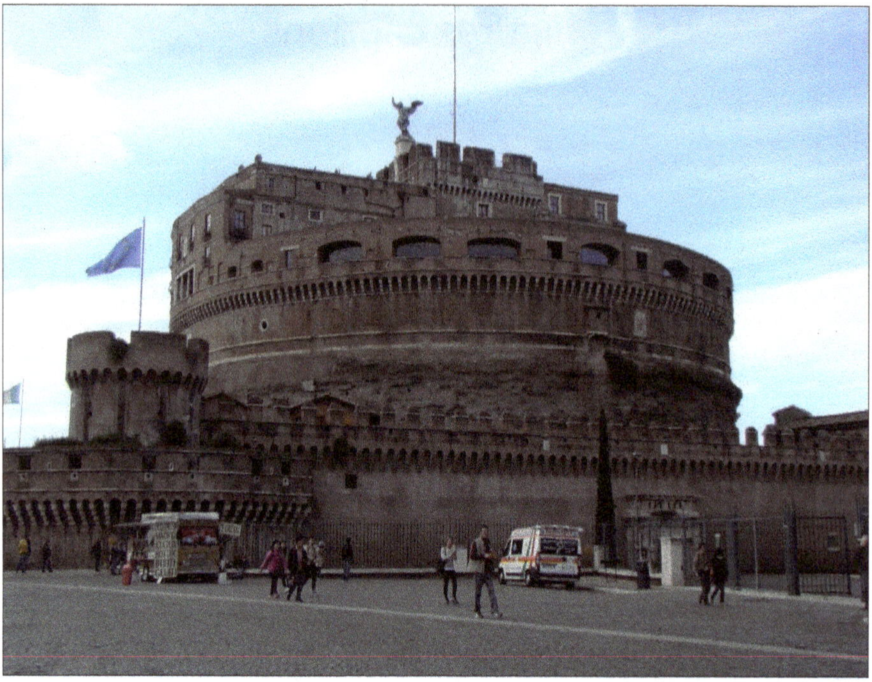

Figure 2. *Mausoleum of Hadrian* (c. 123 AD), Rome, Barbara Bojdo (2016)

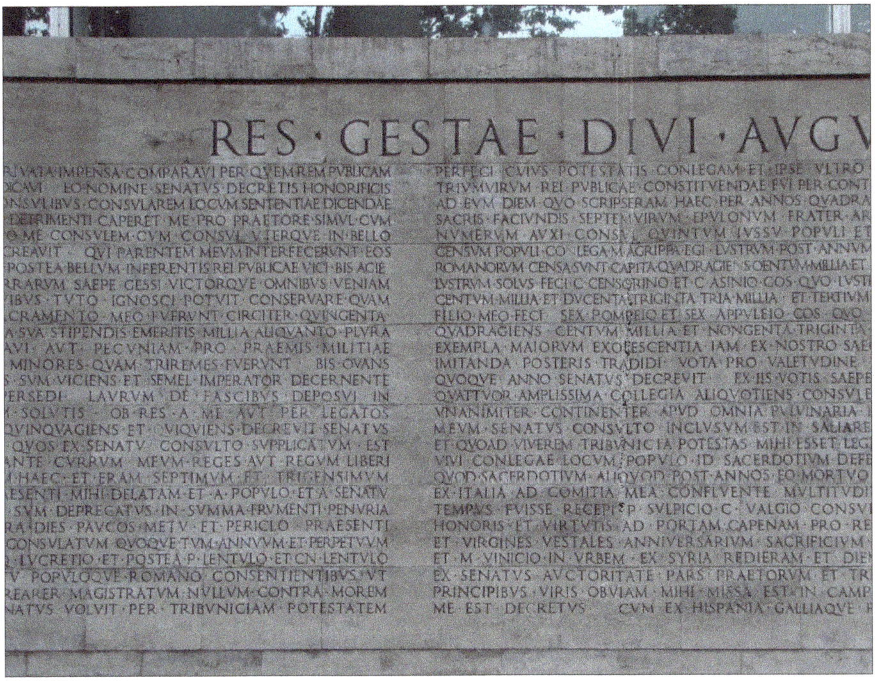

Figure 3. *Res Gestae Divi Augusti* (c. 14 AD), copy of inscription from exterior wall of Museo dell'Ara Pacis, Rome, Barbara Bojdo (2015)

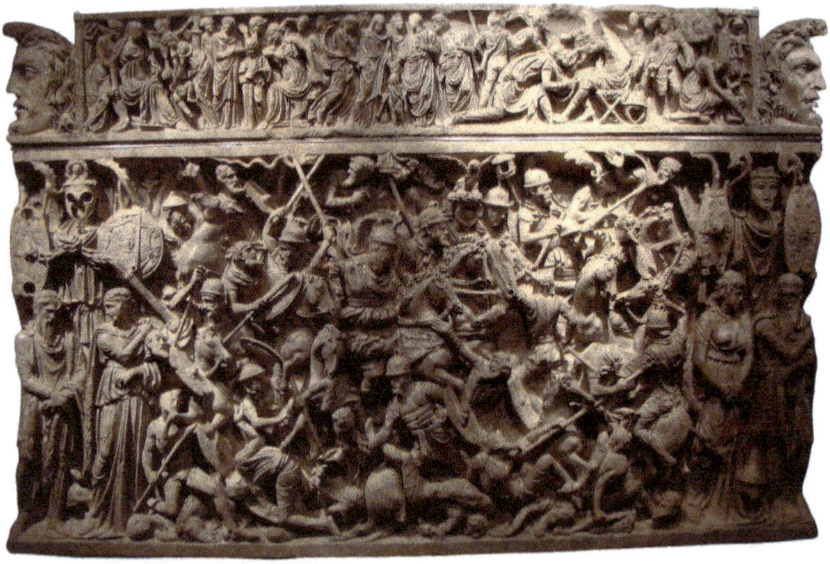

Figure 4. *Portonaccio sarcophagus* (c. 200 AD), Museo Nazionale Romano—Palazzo Massimo alle Terme, Rome, Barbara Bojdo (2016)

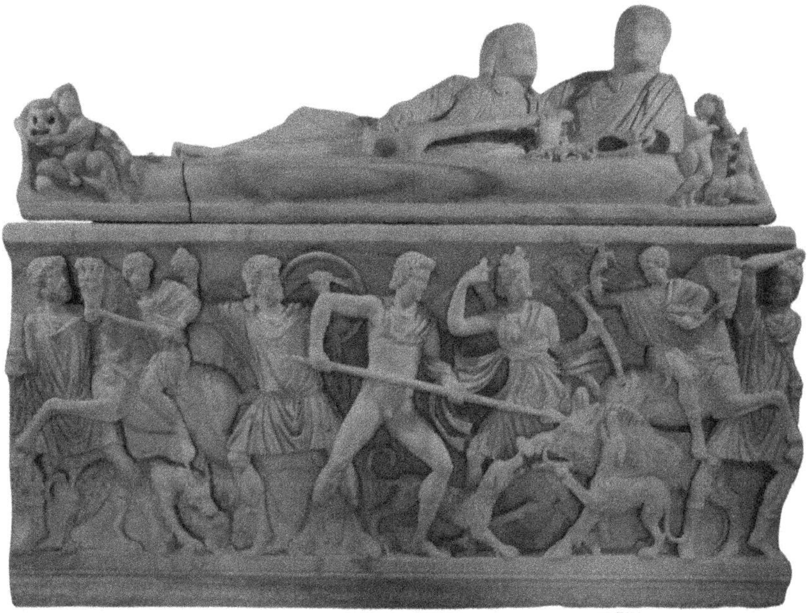

Figure 5. *Attic sarcophagus with scenes depicting life of Achilles—Calydonian Hunt* (c. 200 AD), Musei Capitolini, Rome, Barbara Bojdo (2016)

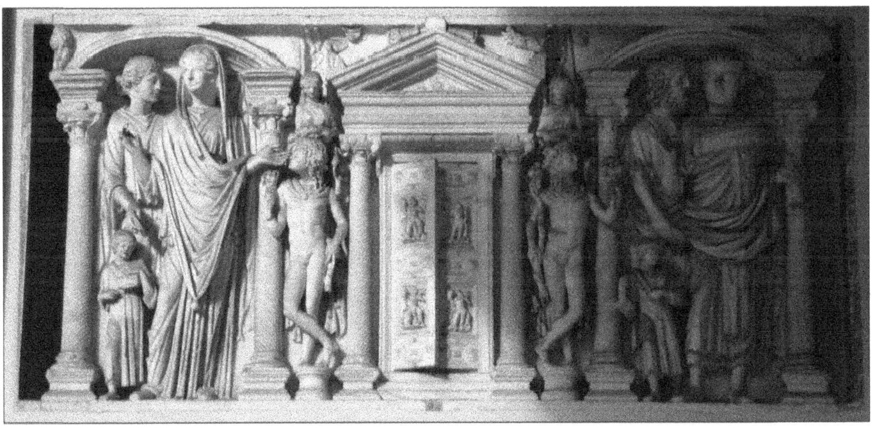

Figure 6. *Front panel from sarcophagus of married couple with door to afterlife* (c. 240–250 AD), Musei Vaticani—Museo Pio Clementino, Rome, Barbara Bojdo (2015)

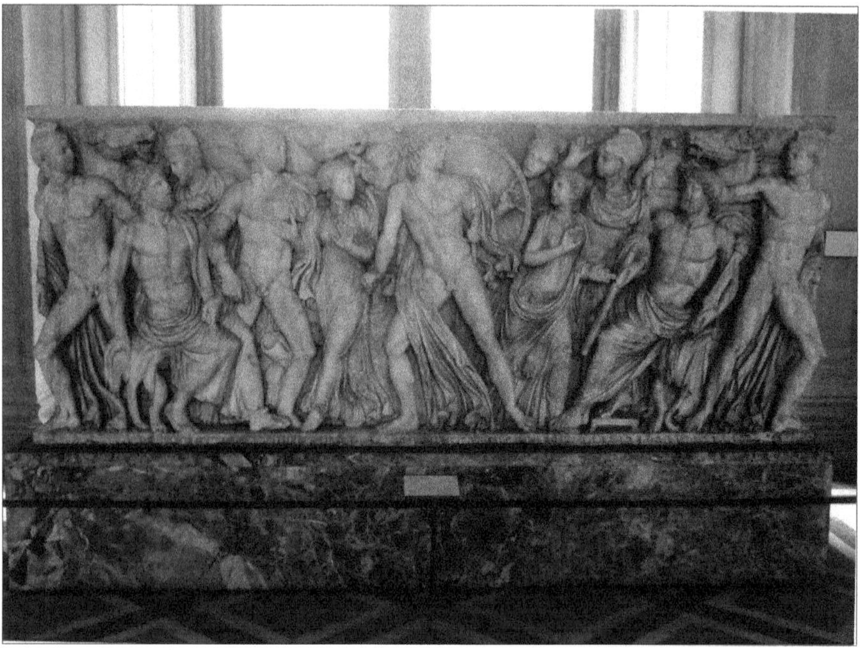

Figure 7. *Attic sarcophagus with scenes depicting life of Achilles* (c. 240 AD), Musée du Louvre, Paris, Barbara Bojdo (2018)

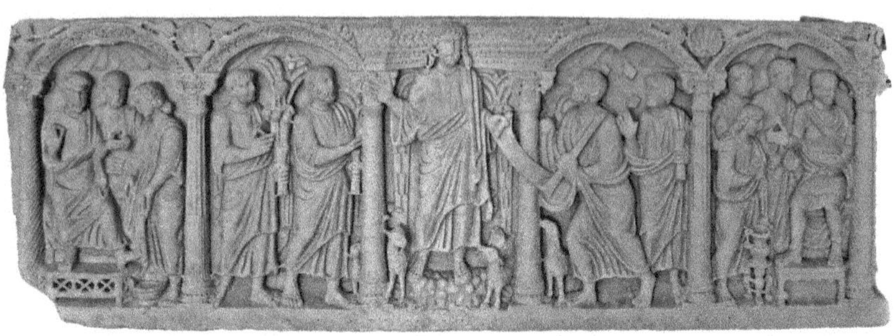

Figure 8. *De la remise de la loi a saint Pierre sarcophagus* (end of 4th c.), Musée departamental de l'Arles antique, Arles, Barbara Bojdo (2012)

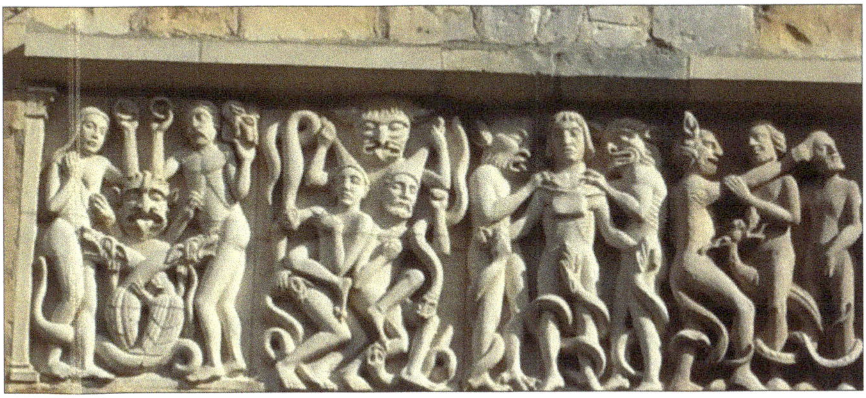

Figure 9. *Romanesque Frieze* (c. 1140), Blessed Virgin Mary Cathedral, Lincoln, Barbara Bojdo (2009)

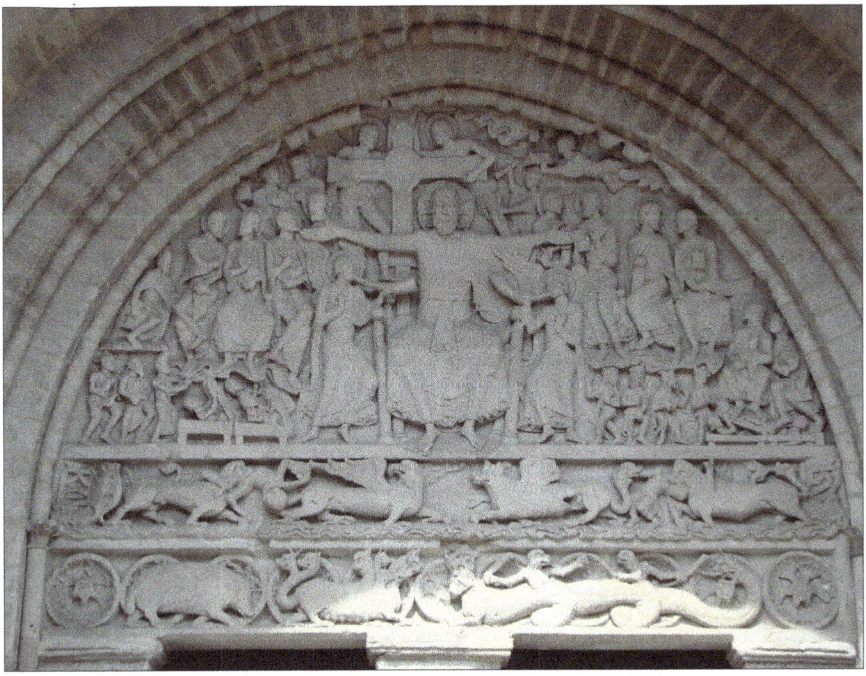

Figure 10. *Tympanum* (c. 1130/c. 1135), Saint Pierre Abbey Church, Baulieu-sur-Dordogne, Barbara Bojdo (2012)

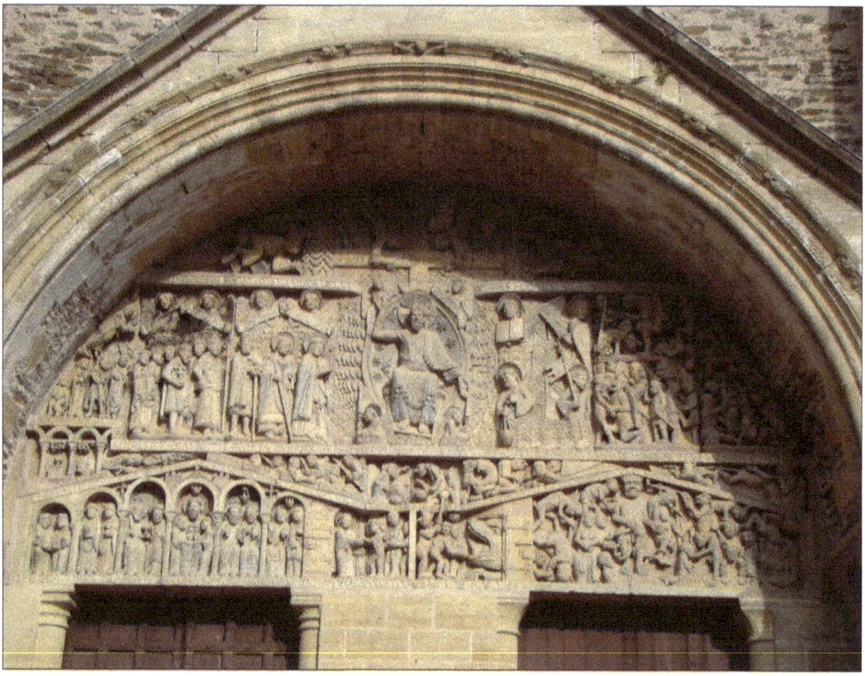

Figure 11. *Tympanum* (c. 1130/c. 1140), Sainte Foy Abbey Church, Congue-en-Rouergue, Barbara Bojdo (2012)

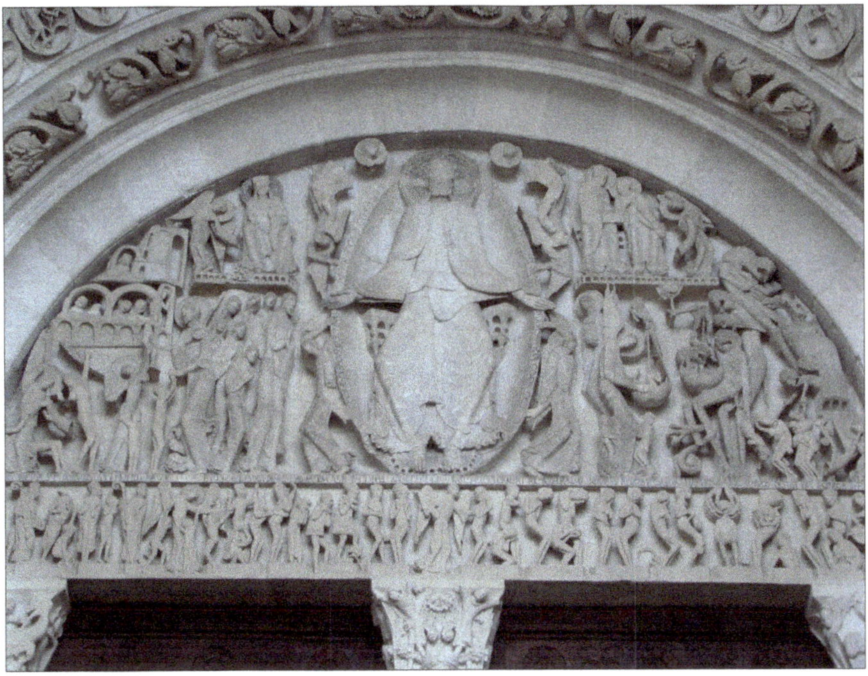

Figure 12. *Tympanum* (after 1125), Sainte Lazare Cathedral, Autun, Barbara Bojdo (2010)

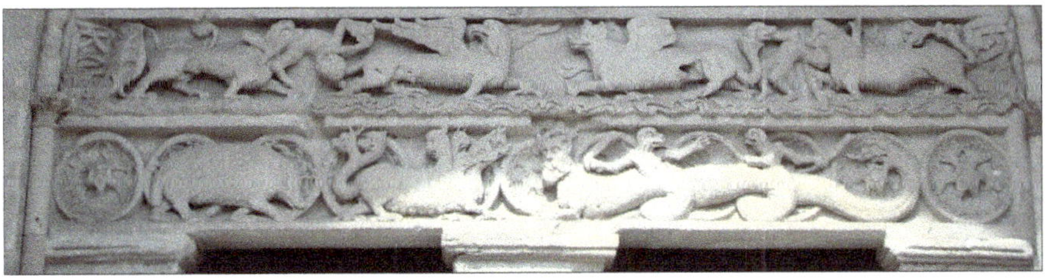

Figure 13. *Tympanum—detail depicting apocaliptic animals and demons* (c. 1130/c. 1135), Saint Pierre Abbey Church, Baulieu-sur-Dordogne, Barbara Bojdo (2012)

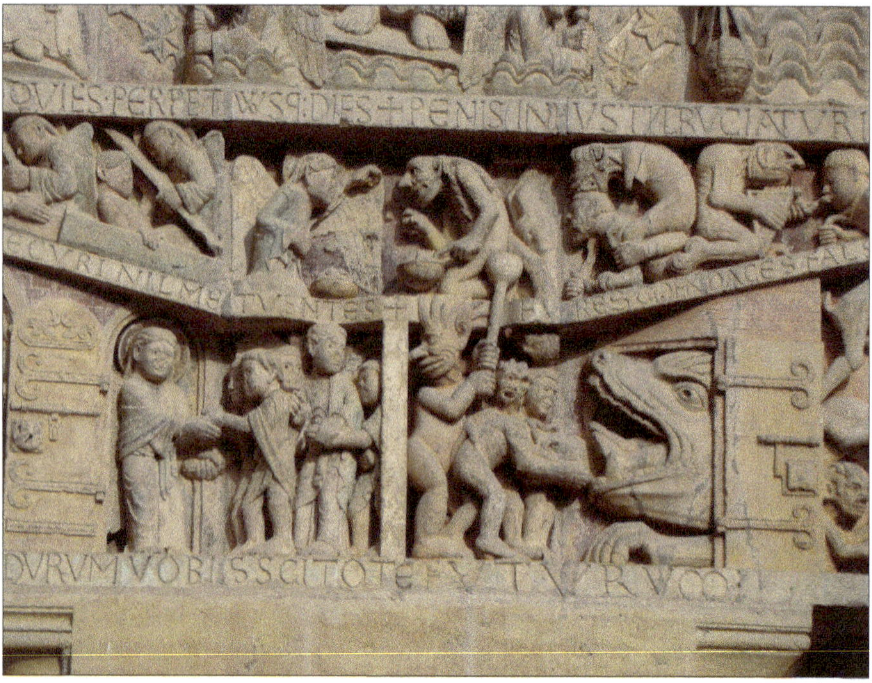

Figure 14. *Tympanum–detail depicting angels and demons* (c. 1130/c. 1140), Sainte Foy Abbey Church, Conque-en-Rouergue, Barbara Bojdo (2012)

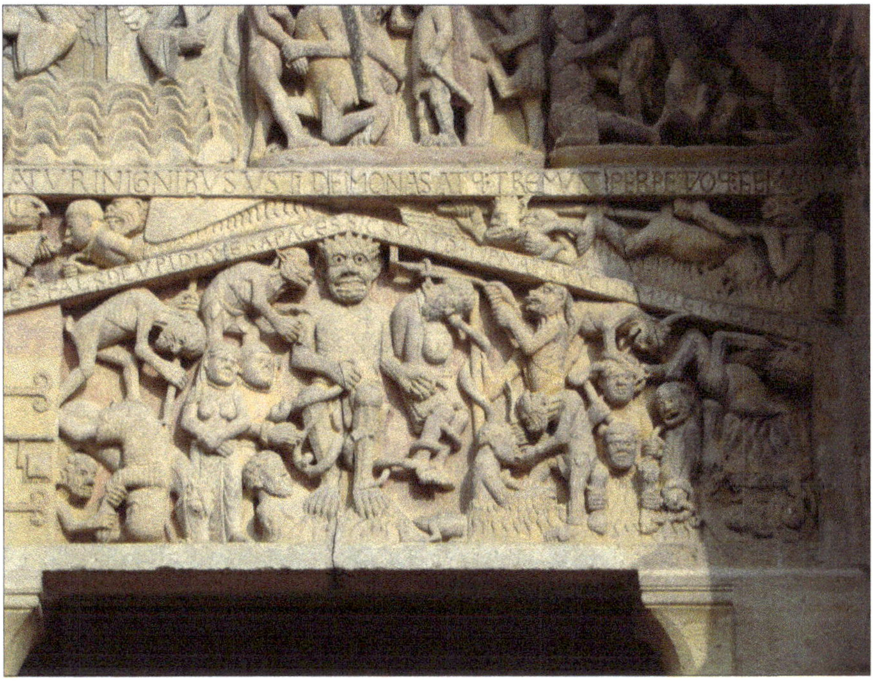

Figure 15. *Tympanum—detail depicting demons, devils and the damned* (c. 1130/c. 1140), Sainte Foy Abbey Church, Conque-en-Rouergue, Barbara Bojdo (2012)

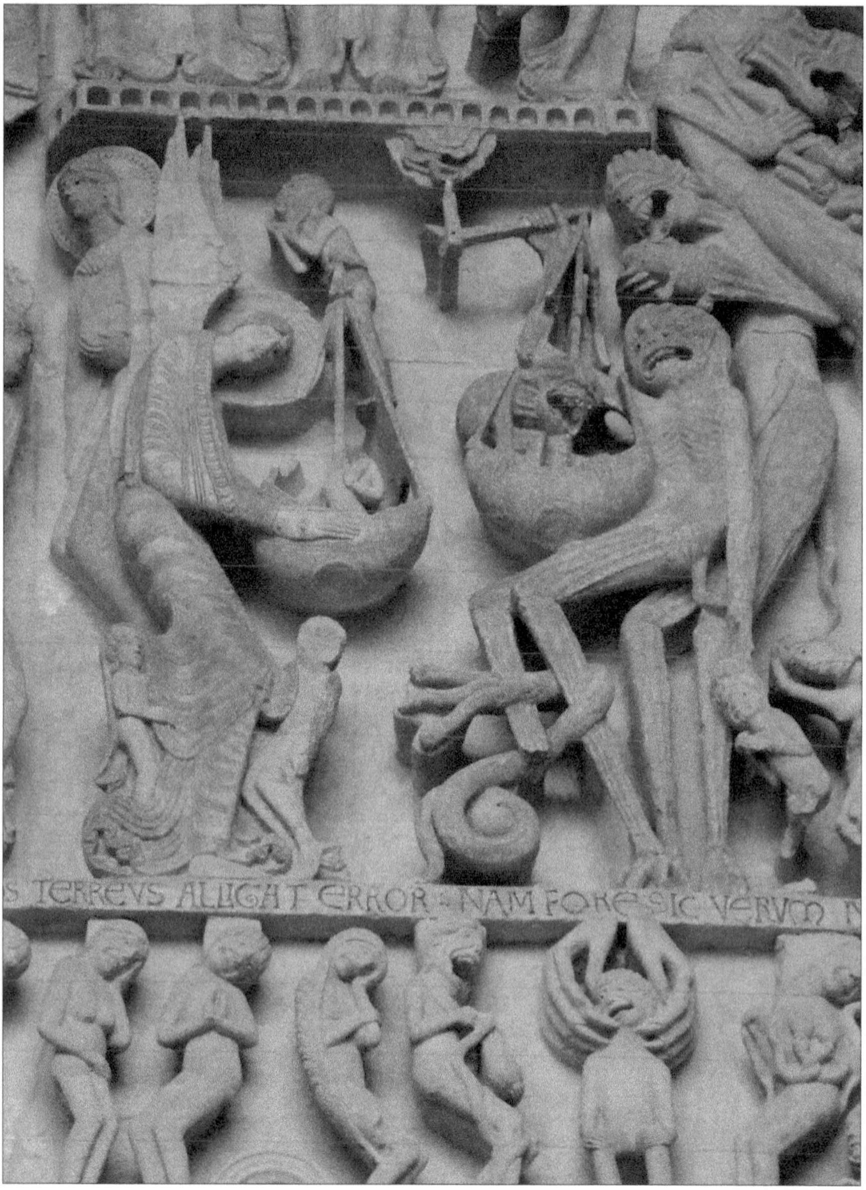

Figure 16. *Tympanum—detail depicting brewing of the souls* (after 1125), Sainte Lazare Cathedral, Autun, Barbara Bojdo (2010)

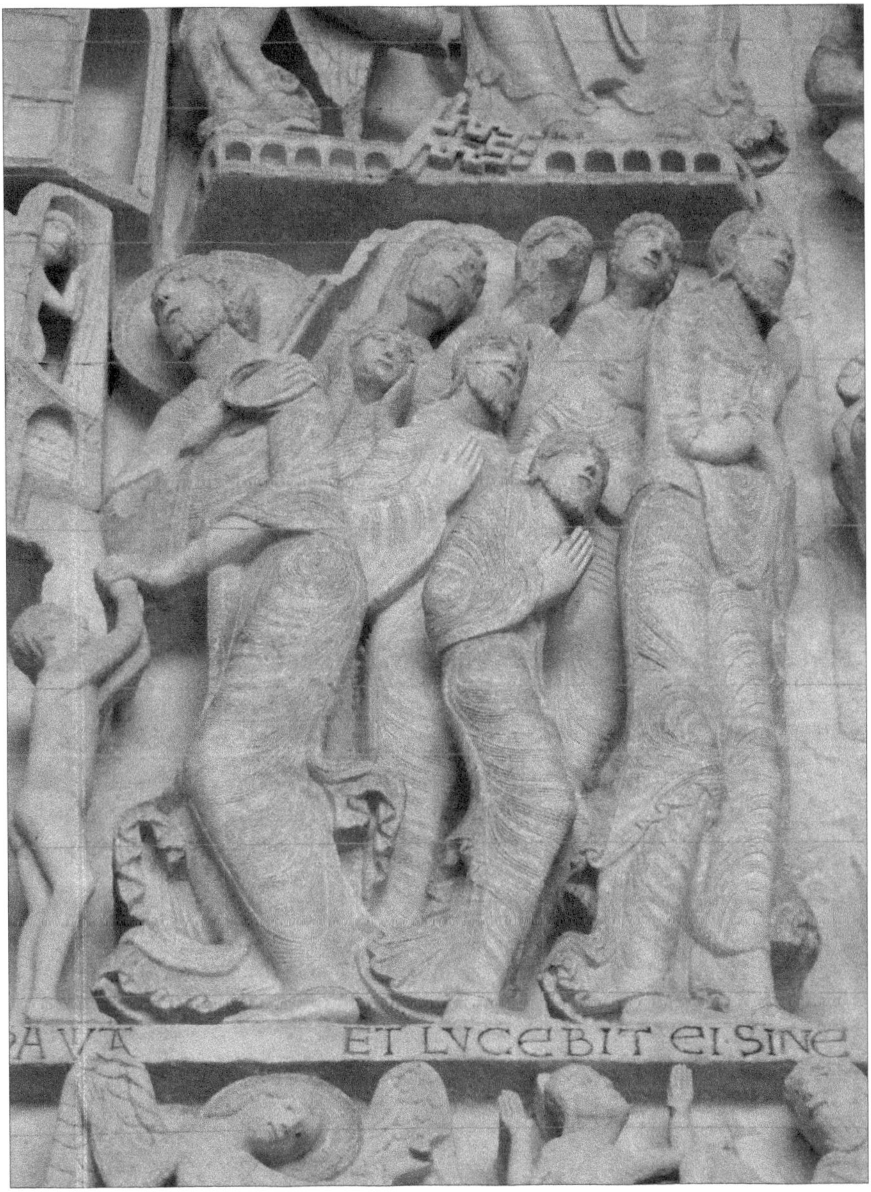

Figure 17. *Tympanum–detail depicting haeven* (after 1125), Sainte Lazare Cathedral, Autun, Barbara Bojdo (2010)

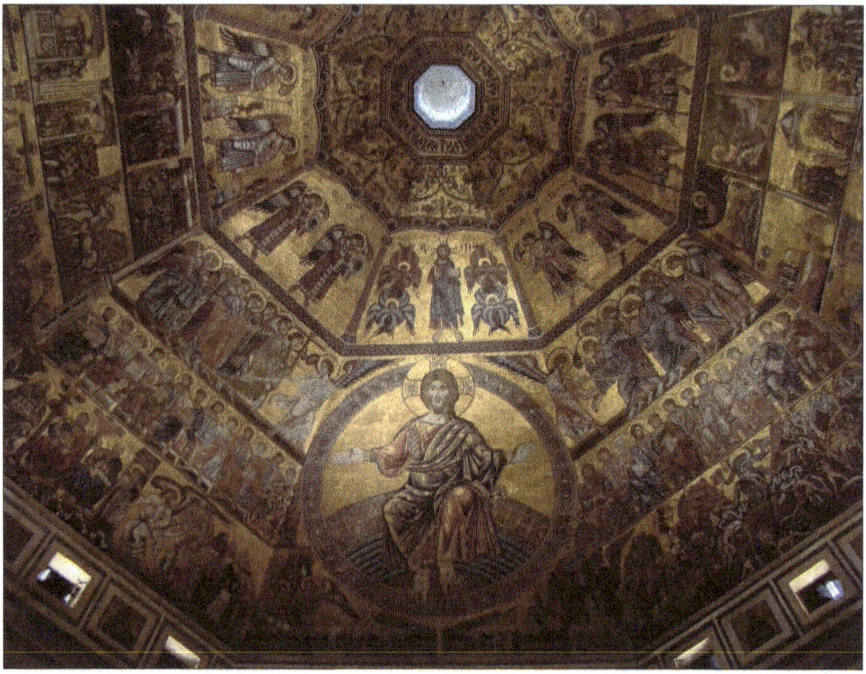

Figure 18. *Last Judgement* (13 th c.), San Giovanni Baptistery, Florence, Barbara Bojdo (2015).

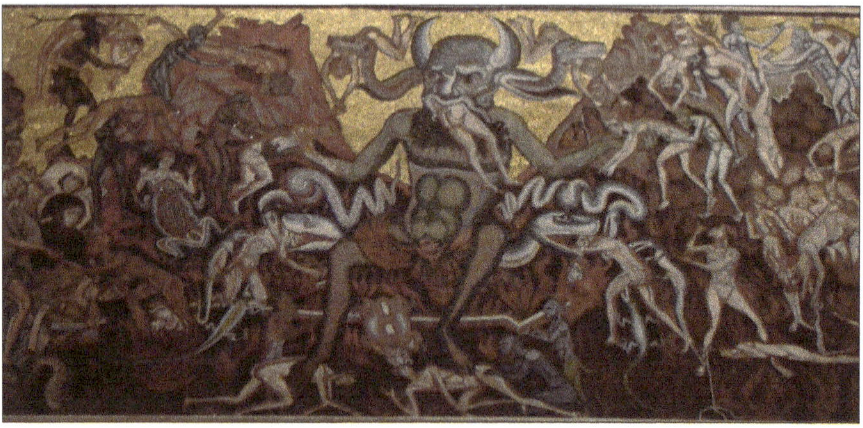

Figure 19. *Last Judgement–detail depicting hellish abyss* (13th c.), San Giovanni Baptistery, Florence, Barbara Bojdo (2015)

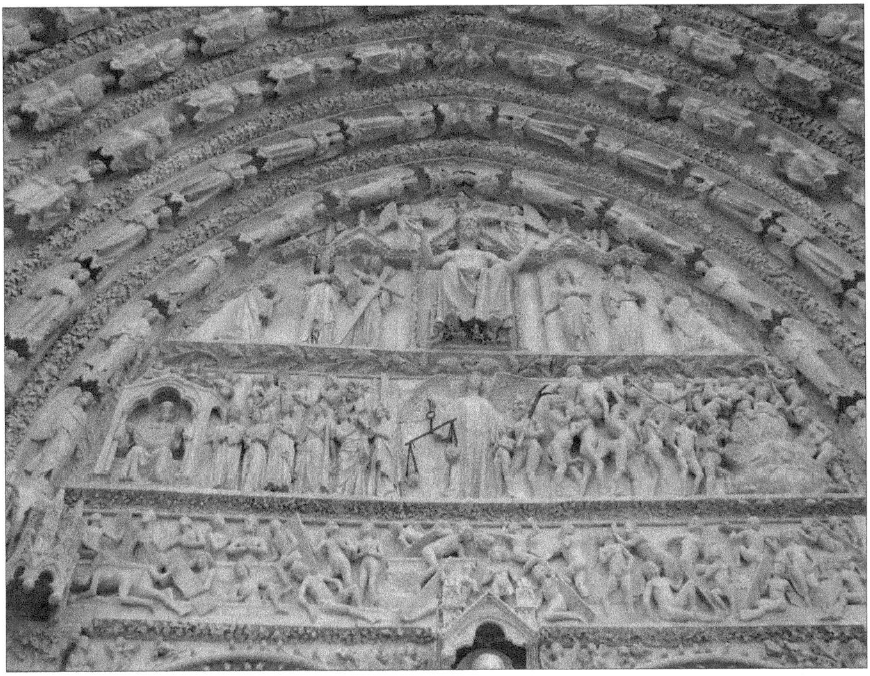

Figure 20. *Tympanum* (13th c.), Saint Étienne Cathedral, Bourges, Barbara Bojdo (2012)

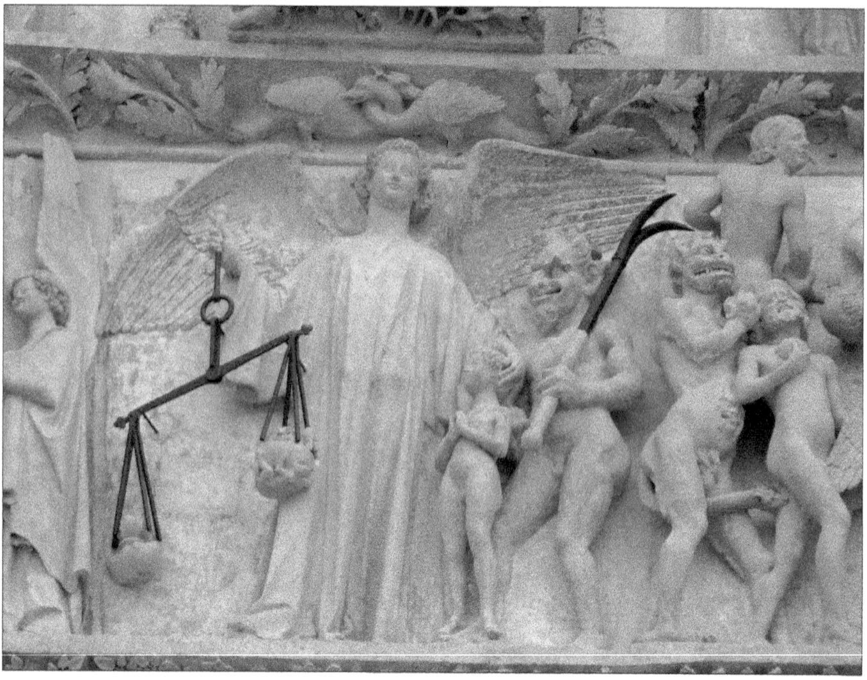

Figure 21. *Tympanum–detail depicting brewing of the souls* (13th c.), Saint Étienne Cathedral, Bourges, Barbara Bojdo (2012)

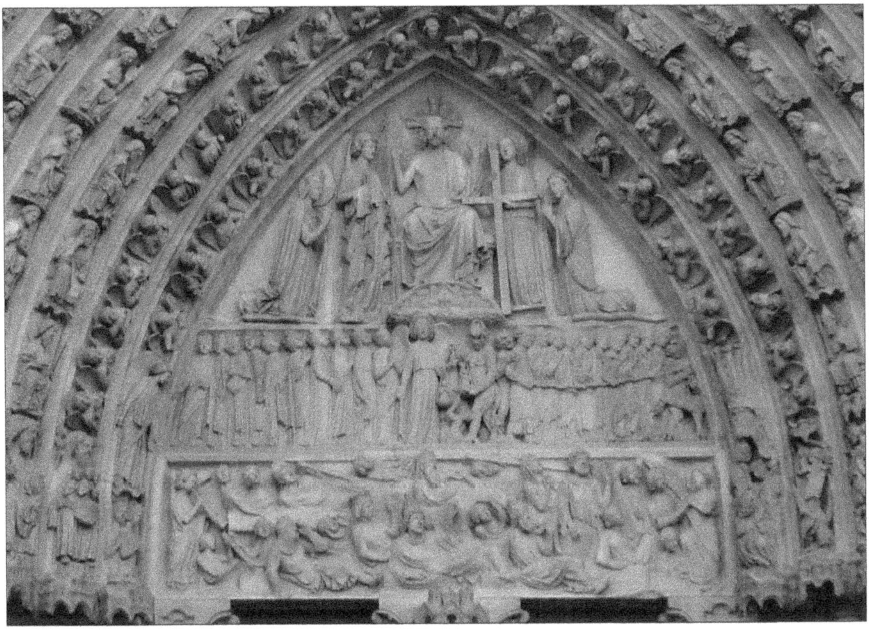

Figure 22. *Tympanum* (13th c.), Notre Dame Cathedral, Paris, Barbara Bojdo (2018)

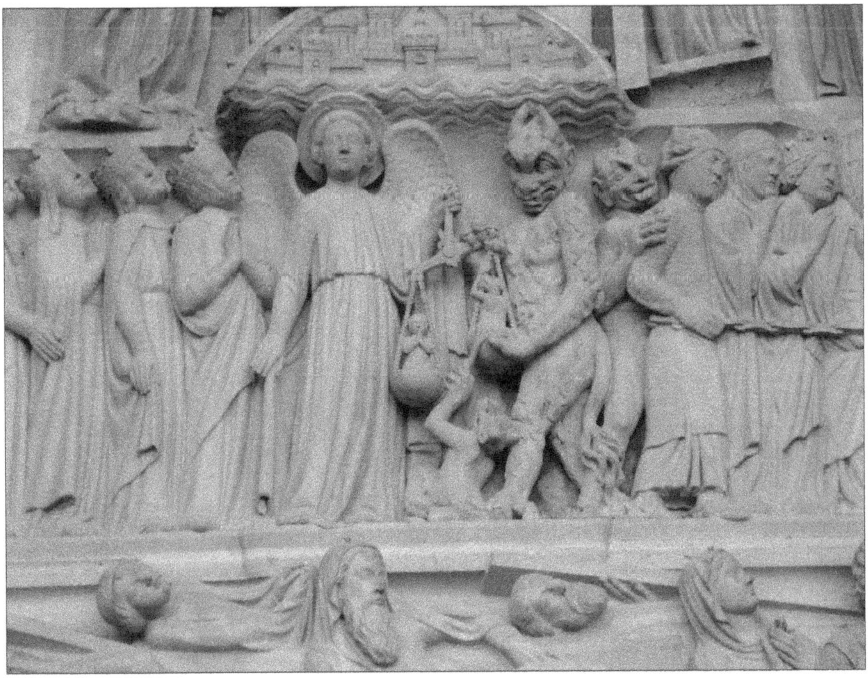

Figure 23. *Tympanum—detail depicting brewing of the souls* (13th c.), Notre Dame Cathedral, Paris, Barbara Bojdo (2018)

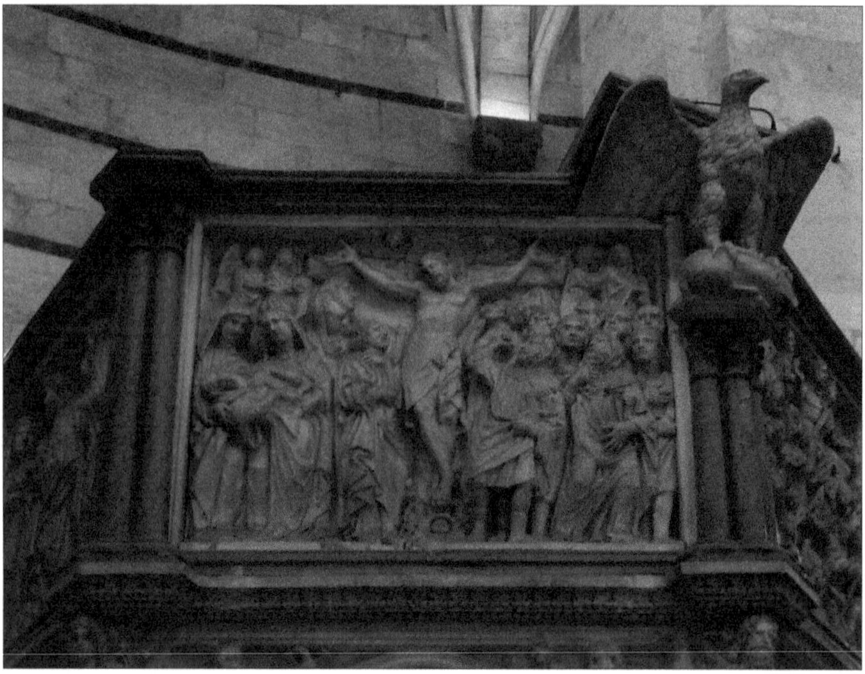

Figure 24. Nicolo Pisano 1260, *Crucifiction–panel from pulpit*, San Giovanni Baptistery, Piza, Barbara Bojdo (2015)

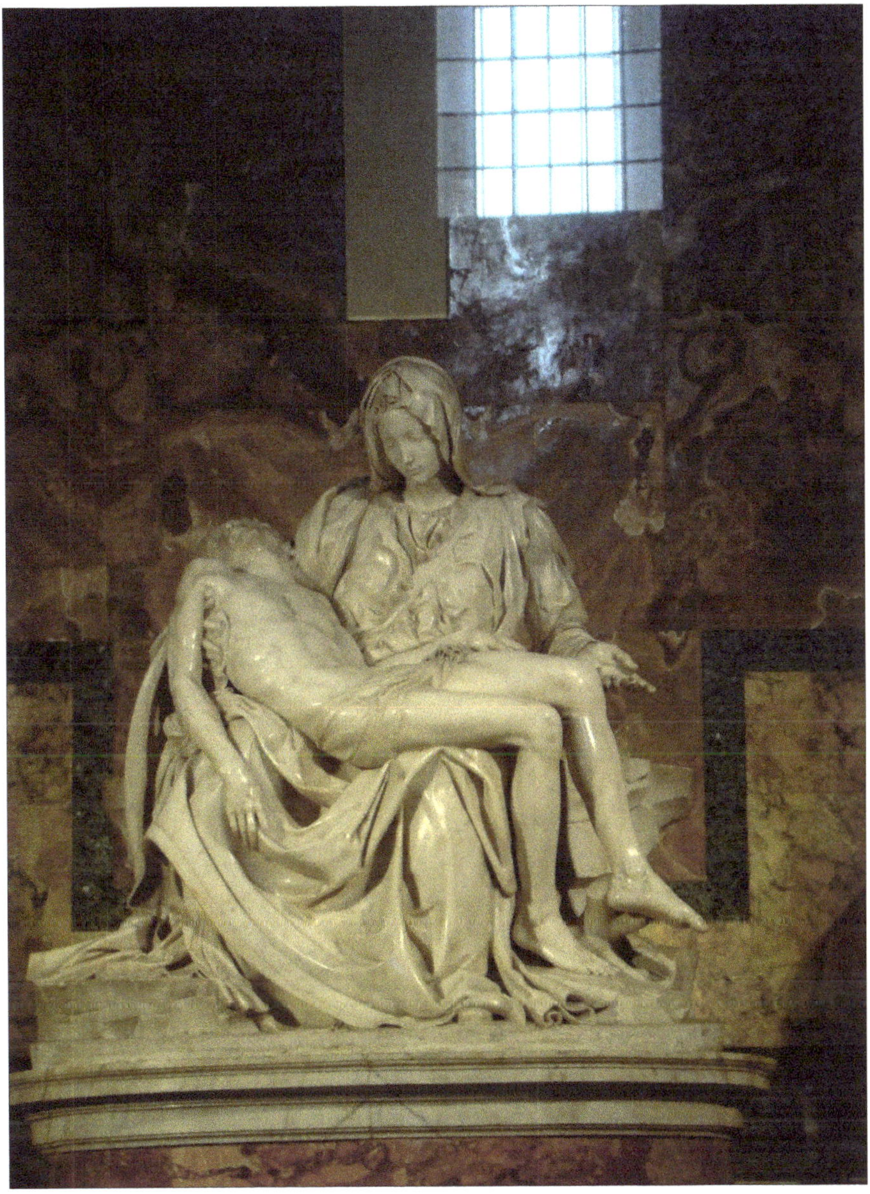

Figure 25. Michelangelo Buonarotti 1498–1506, *Pietà*, San Pietro Basilica, Vatican City, Barbara Bojdo (2015)

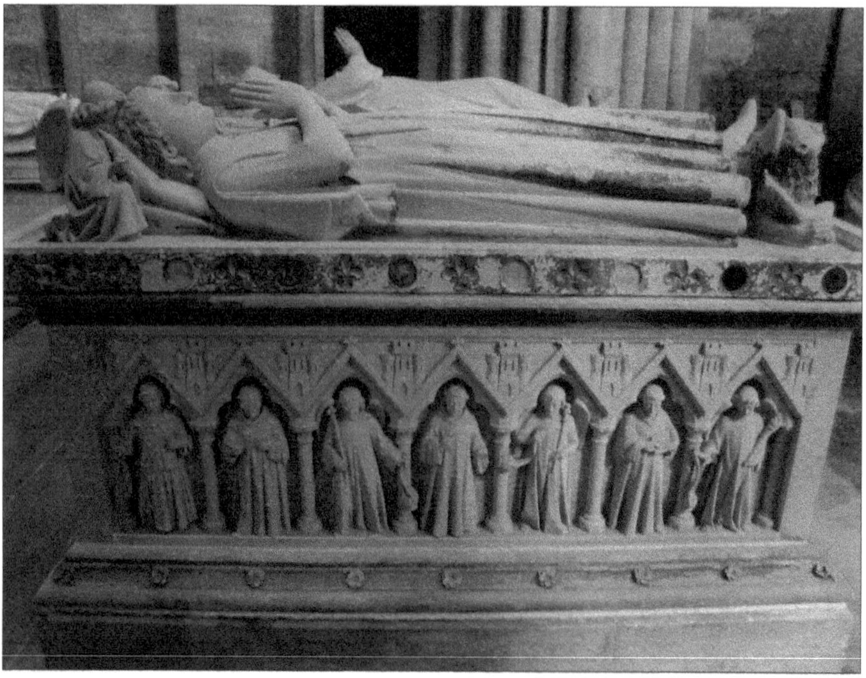

Figure 26. *Gisant tomb of Philip de France* (d. 1285), Saint Denis Cathedral, Paris, Barbara Bojdo (2018).

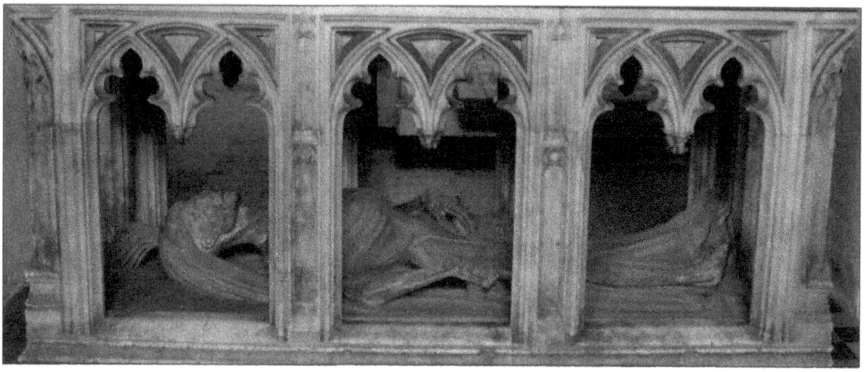

Figure 27. *Cadaver of John FitzAlan* (d. 1435), Arundel Castel, Arundel, Barbara Bojdo (2009)

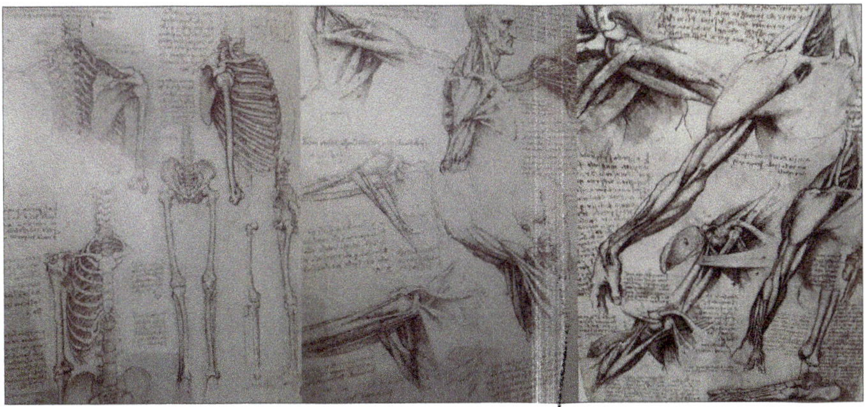

Figure 28. Leonardo da Vinci about 1485 to 1510–1515, *Anatomical sketches reproductions*, Museo Leonardo da Vinci, Florence, Barbara Bojdo (2017)

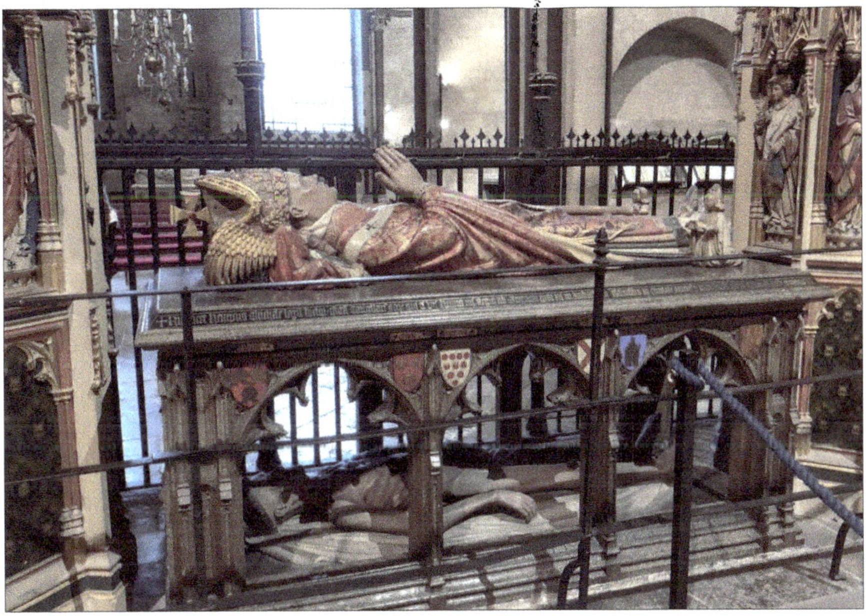

Figure 29. *Tomb of Archbishop Henry Chichele* (d. 1443), Cathedral and Metropolitical Church of Christ, Canterbury, Barbara Bojdo (2006)

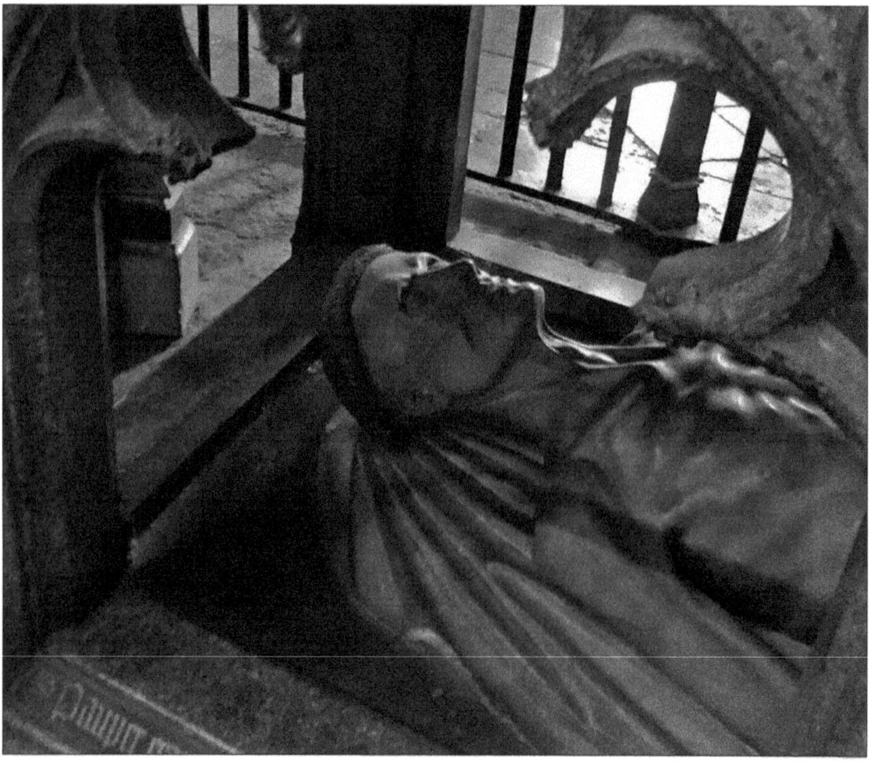

Figure 30. *Transi of Archbishop Henry Chichele–detail* (d. 1443), Cathedral and Metropolitical Church of Christ, Canterbury, Barbara Bojdo (2006)

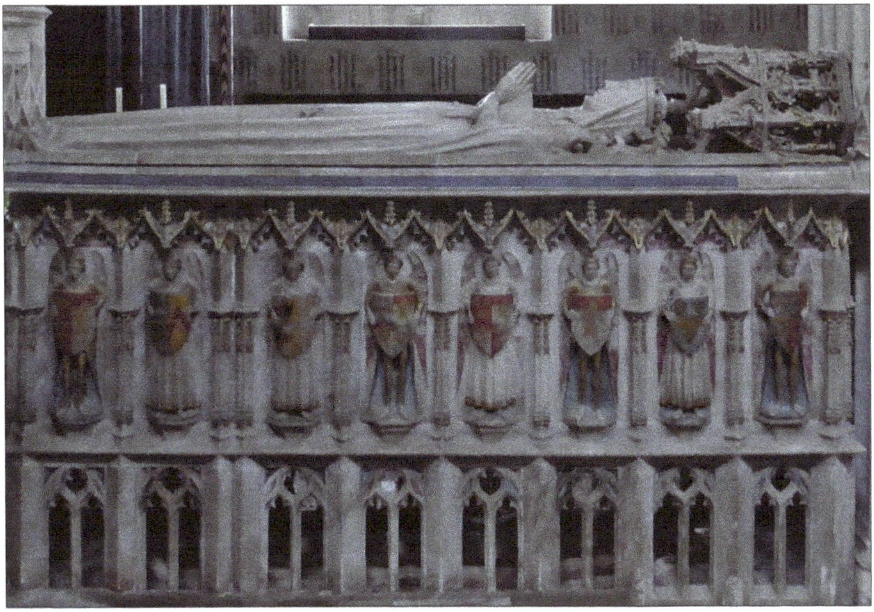

Figure 31. *Tomb of Alice de la Pole* (d. 1475), Saint Mary the Virgin Church, Ewelme, Barbara Bojdo (2006)

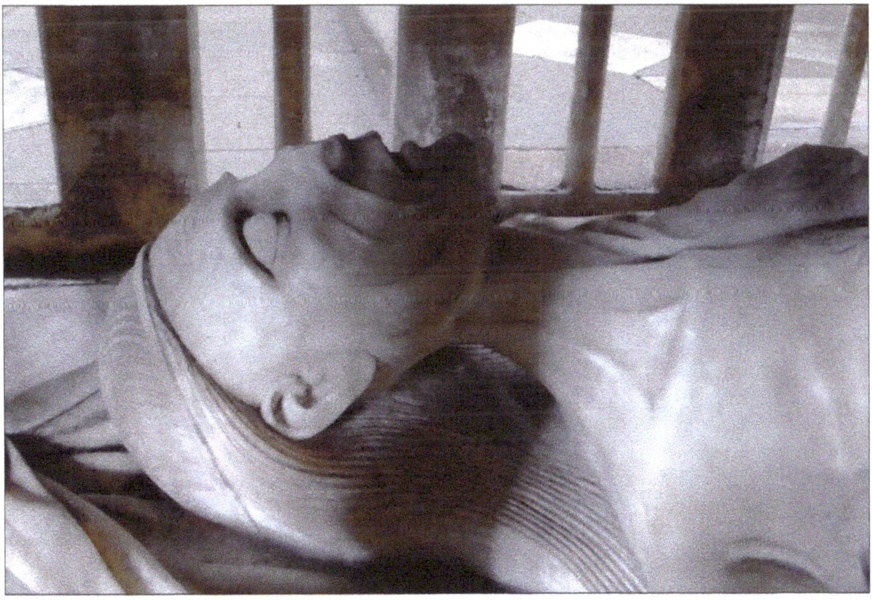

Figure 32. *Tomb of Alice de la Pole–detail* (d. 1475), Saint Mary the Virgin Church, Ewelme, Barbara Bojdo (2006)

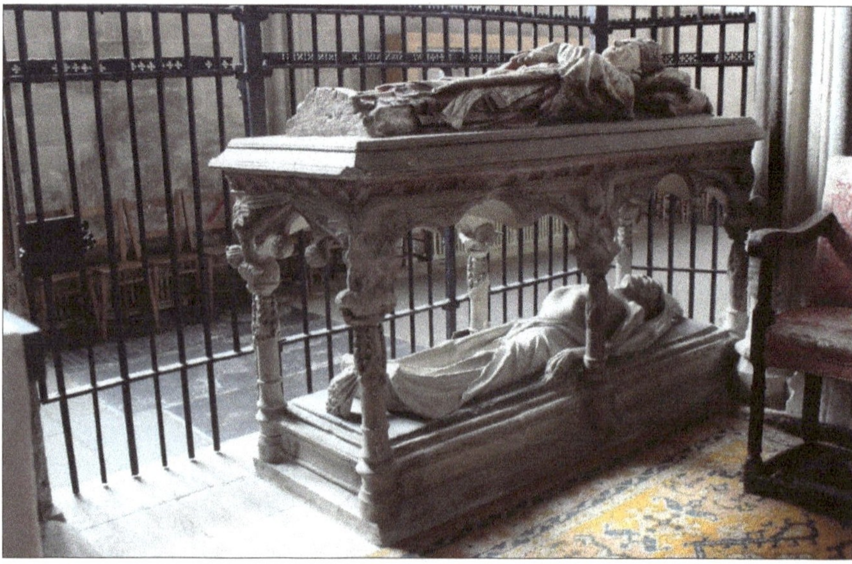

Figure 33. *Tomb of Bishop Thomas Bekington* (d. 1450–1451), Saint Andrew Cathedral, Wells, Barbara Bojdo (2008)

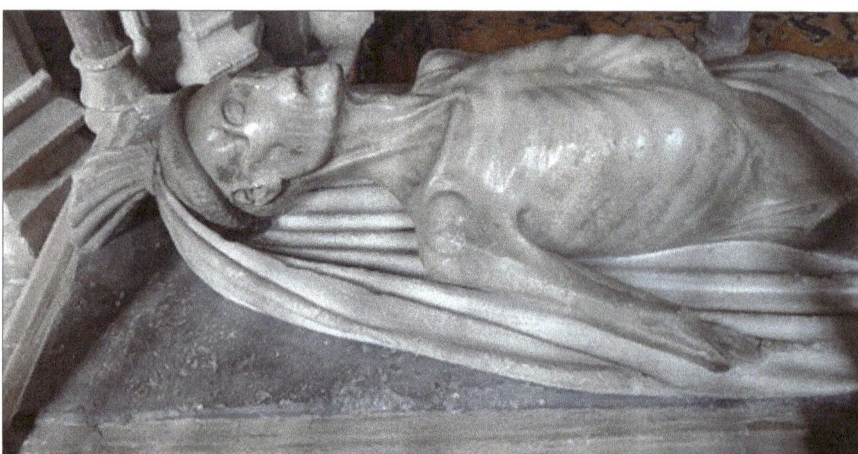

Figure 34. *Transi of Bishop Thomas Bekington—detail* (d. 1450–1451), Saint Andrew Cathedral, Wells, Barbara Bojdo (2008)

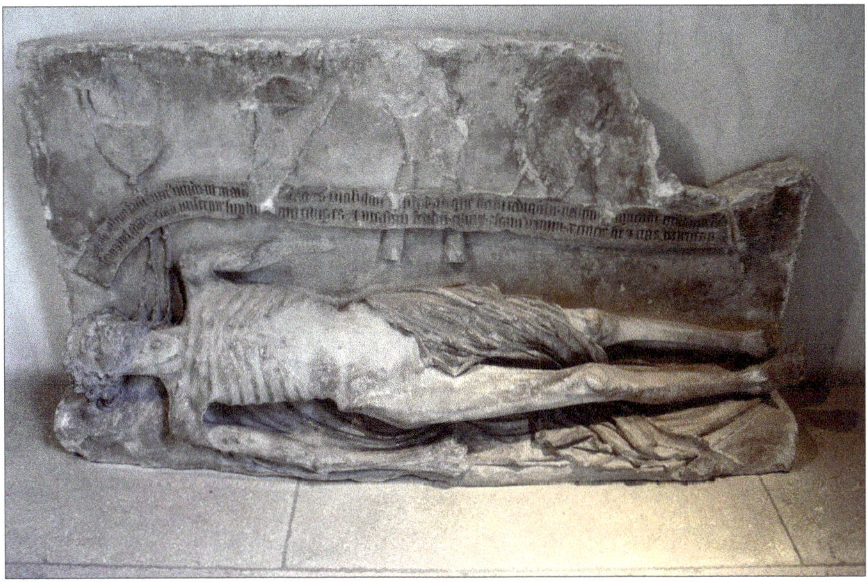

Figure 35. *Transi of Cardinal Jean de La Grange* (d. 1402), Musée du Petit Palais, Avignon, Barbara Bojdo (2012)

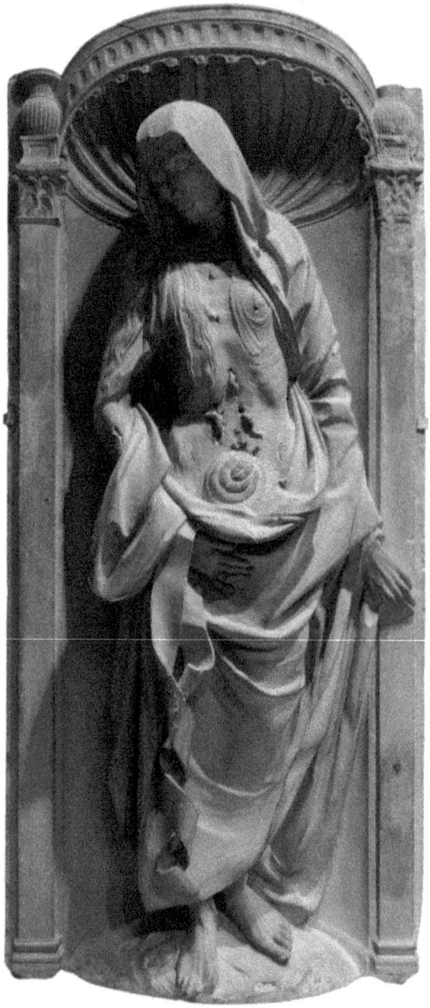

Figure 36. *Sculpture in transi type of Jeanne de Burbon-Vendôme* (d. 1521), Musée du Louvre, Paris, Barbara Bojdo (2018)

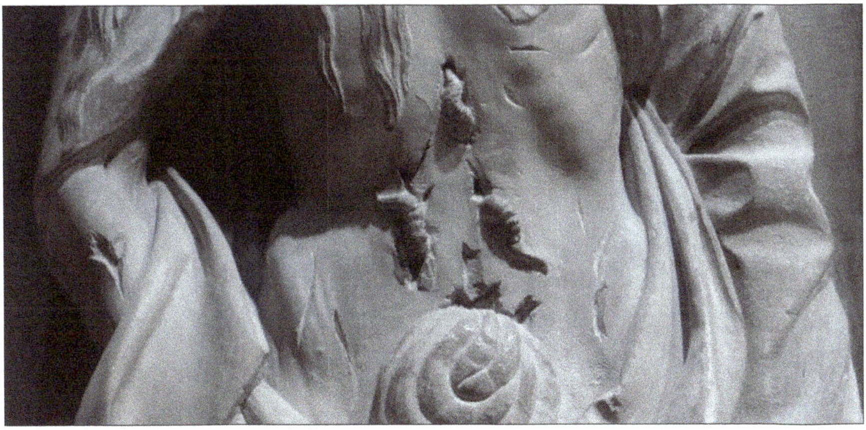

Figure 37. *Sculpture in transi type of Jeanne de Burbon-Vendôme—detail* (d. 1521), Musée du Louvre, Paris, Barbara Bojdo (2018)

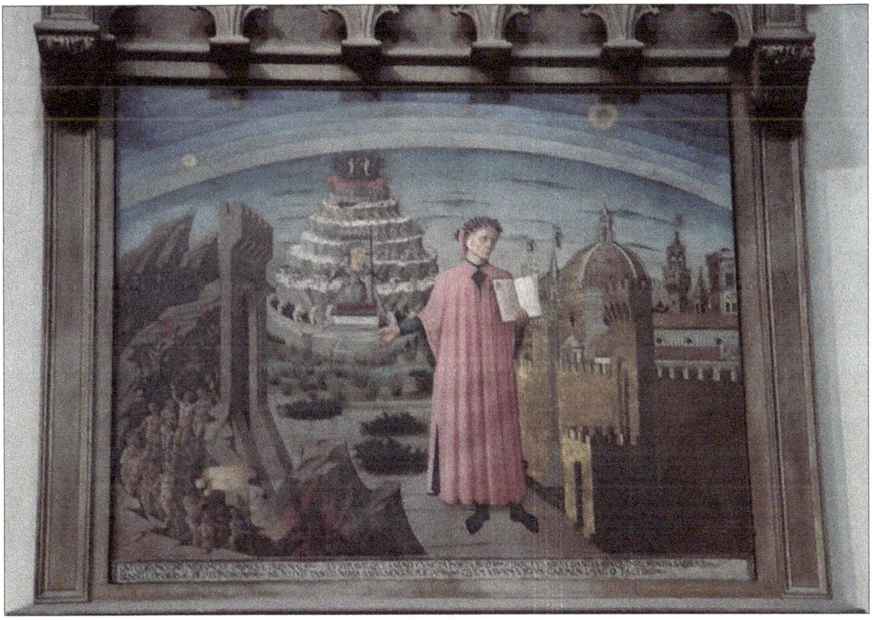

Figure 38. Domenico di Michelino 1465, *La Divina Commedia illumina Firenze*, Santa Maria del Fiore Cathedral, Florence, Barbara Bojdo (2015)

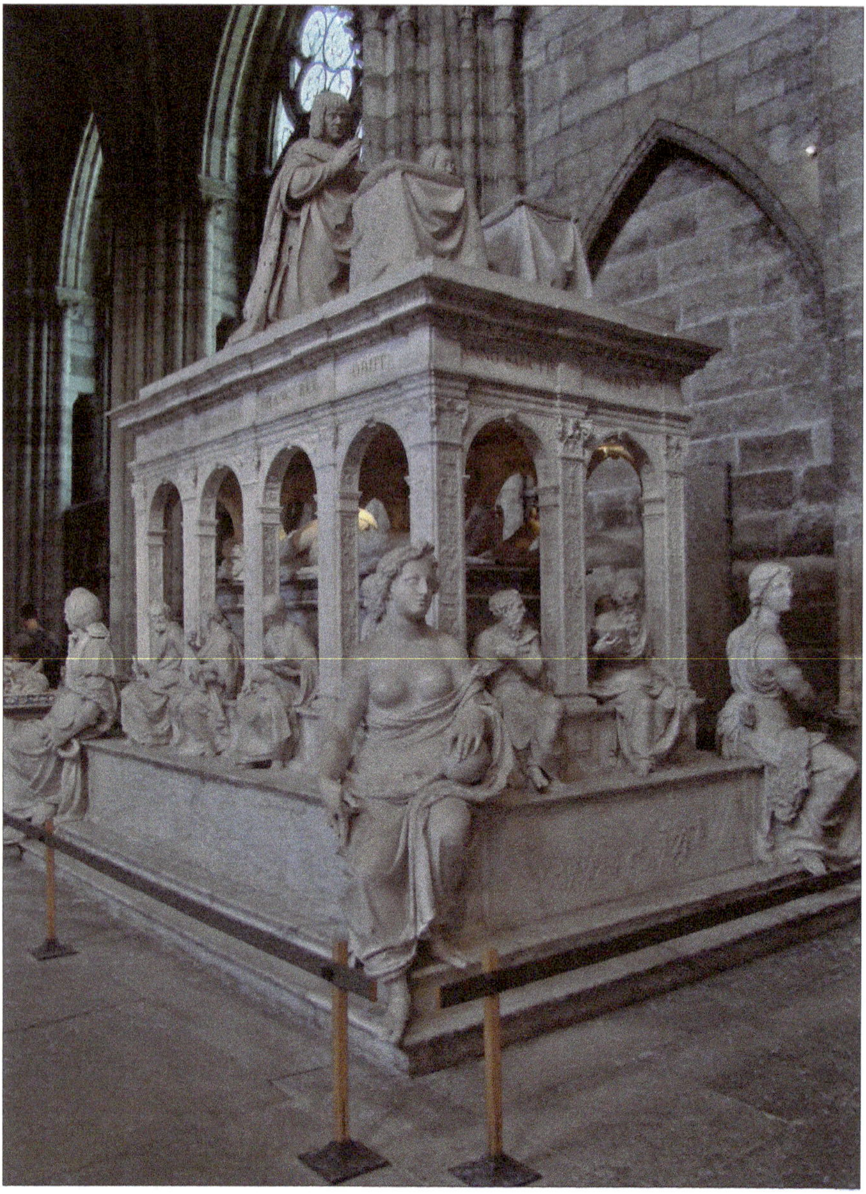

Figure 39. Antonio & Giovanni Giusti 1515–1531, *Tomb of King Louis XII and Anne of Bretagne*, Saint Denis Cathedral, Paris, Barbara Bojdo (2018)

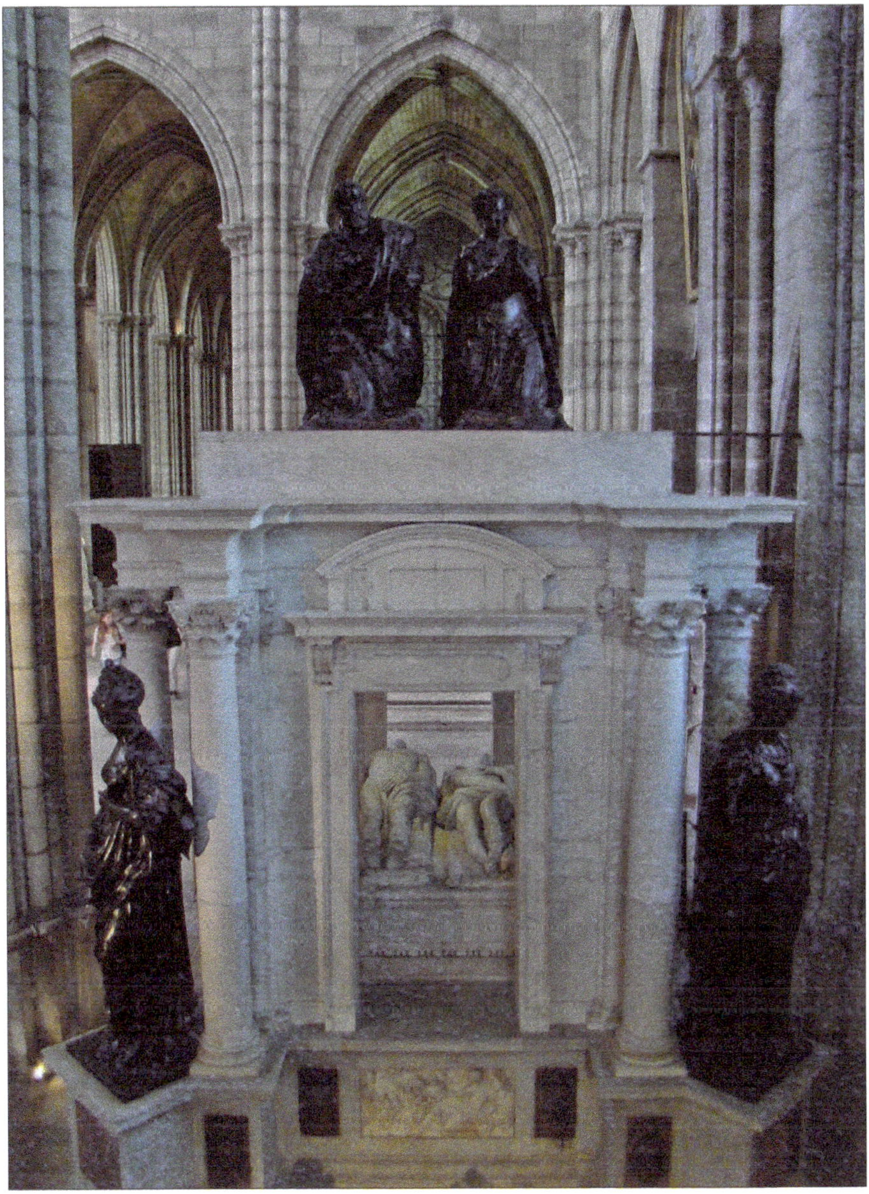

Figure 40. G. Pilon & J. Ponce 1560–1573, *Tomb of King Henry II and Catherine de' Medici*, Saint Denis Cathedral, Paris, Barbara Bojdo (2018)

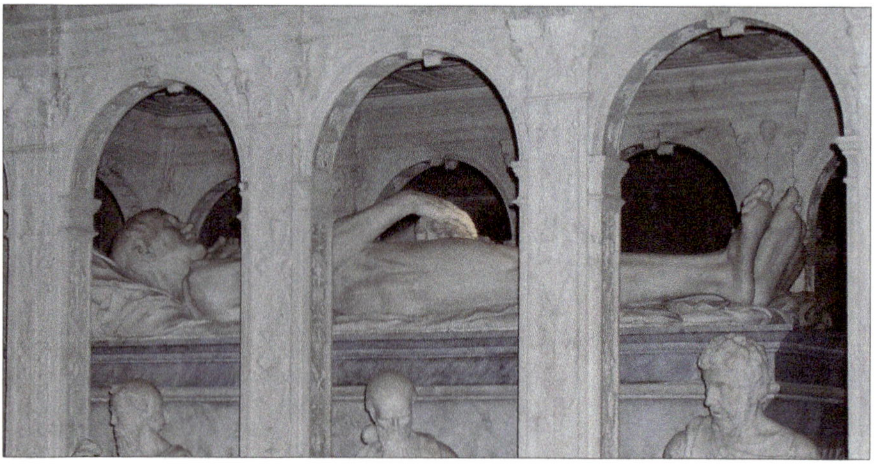

Figure 41. Antonio & Giovanni Giusti 1515–1531, *Transi of King Louis XII and Anne of Bretagne*, Saint Denis Cathedral, Paris, Barbara Bojdo (2018)

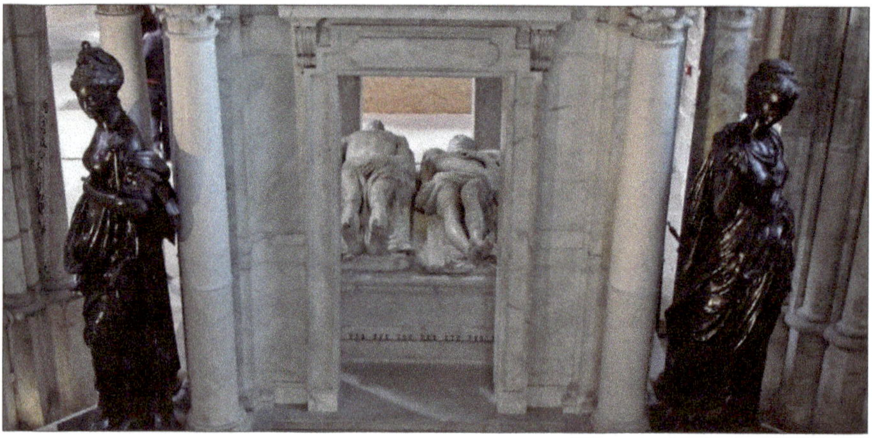

Figure 42. G. Pilon & J. Ponce 1560–1573, *Transi of King Henry II and Catherine de' Medici*, Saint Denis Cathedral, Paris, Barbara Bojdo (2018)

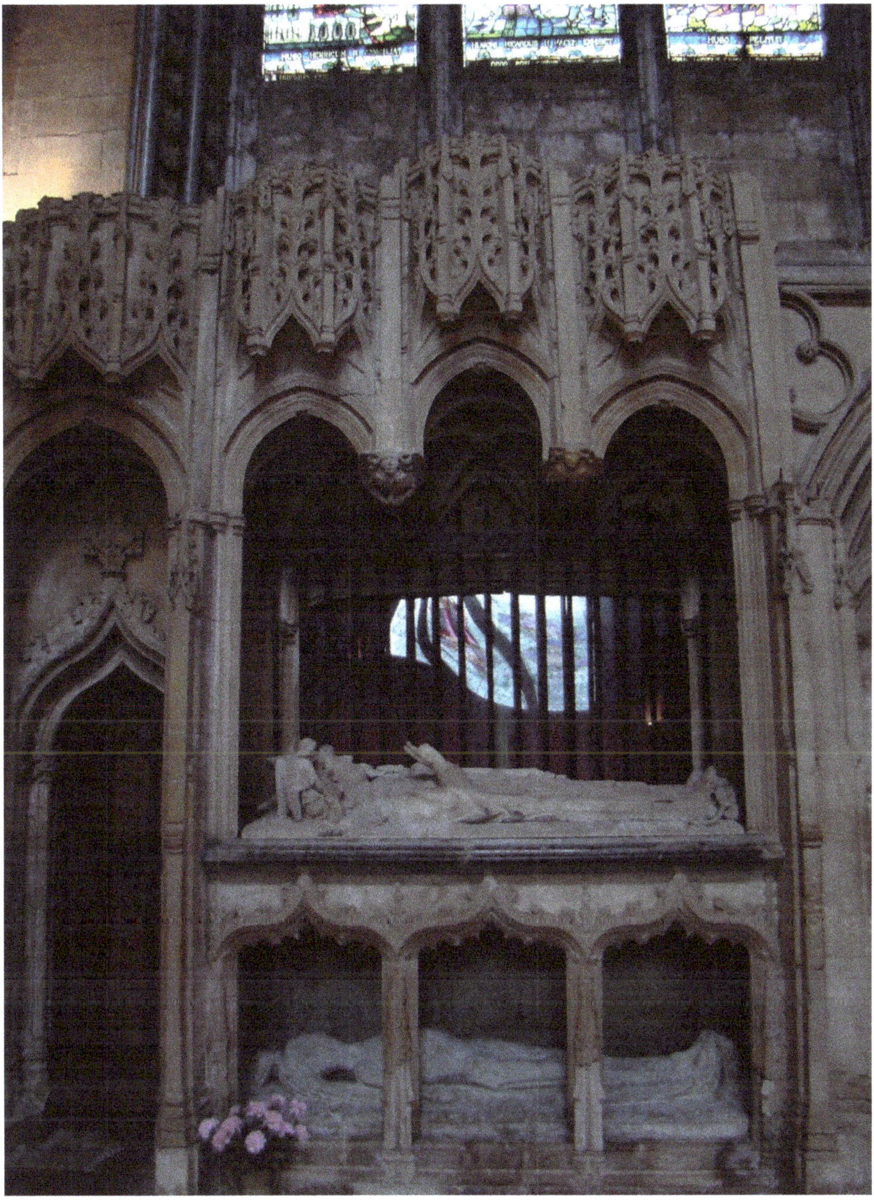

Figure 43. *Tomb of Richard Fleming* (d. 1431), Blessed Virgin Mary Cathedral, Lincoln, Barbara Bojdo (2009)

Index of names

Subject index

Managing editor
Zofia Sajdek

Language editor
Renata Włodek

Proofreading
Tomasz P. Bocheński / WIELE KROPEK

Typesetting
Wojciech Wojewoda

Jagiellonian University Press
Editorial Offices: Michałowskiego 9/2, 31-126 Kraków
Phone: +48 12 663 23 80

GPSR Authorized Representative: Easy Access System Europe, Mustamäe tee 50, 10621 Tallinn, Estonia, gpsr.requests@easproject.com

www.ingramcontent.com/pod-product-compliance
Ingram Content Group UK Ltd.
Pitfield, Milton Keynes, MK11 3LW, UK
UKHW020033140626
472189UK00004B/213
* 9 7 8 8 3 2 3 3 5 0 5 5 2 *